SIMON & SCHUSTER'S POCKET GUIDE TO

WILDERNESS MEDICINE

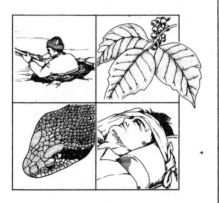

Paul G. Gill, Jr., M.D.

A Fireside Book
Published by Simon & Schuster
New York London Toronto Sydney
Tokyo Singapore

Fireside
Simon & Schuster Building
Rockefeller Center
1230 Avenue of the Americas
New York, New York 10020

Copyright © 1991 by Paul G. Gill, Jr.

FIRESIDE and colophon are registered trademarks
of Simon & Schuster Inc.

DESIGNED BY BARBARA MARKS
ILLUSTRATED BY WILLIAM P. HAMILTON

Manufactured in the United States of America

10 9 8 7 6 5 4 3   Pbk.

Library of Congress Cataloging-in-Publication Data
Gill, Paul G., date.
    Simon & Schuster's pocket guide to wilder-
ness medicine / Paul G. Gill, Jr.
        p. cm.
    "A Fireside book."
    Includes index.
    1. Mountaineering—Accidents and injuries—
Handbooks, manuals, etc. 2. First aid in illness
and injury. I. Title. II. Title: Simon and
Schuster's pocket guide to wilderness medicine.
III. Title: Wilderness medicine.
RC1220.M6G55   1991
616.02′52—dc20   90–27523
                                                          CIP

ISBN 0-671-70615-2 Pbk.

Contents

Introduction 4

1. The Basics: Shock, CPR, and the ABCs 7
2. Soft-Tissue Injuries: Sprains, Strains, Cuts, and Bumps 18
3. Burns 28
4. Fractures and Dislocations 34
5. Heads Up: Head and Neck Injuries in the Wild 47
6. Chest and Abdominal Injuries 54
7. Eye, Ear, Nose, and Throat Problems 63
8. Hypothermia 71
9. Frostbite and Other Cold Injuries 81
10. Solar Injuries and Heat Illness 87
11. Lightning Injuries 99
12. Drowning and Near-Drowning 108
13. Insect, Spider, and Scorpion Bites and Stings 115
14. Snake and Reptile Bites 127
15. Plant Dermatitis 136
16. Infectious Diarrhea and Field Water Disinfection 143
17. Motion Sickness 151
18. Rabies, Lyme Disease, and Other Wilderness Infections 156
19. High-Altitude Illness 166
20. Dental Emergencies 171
21. Foot Care in the Wild 176
22. Wilderness Survival 179
23. The Wilderness Medical Kit 187
Index 193

INTRODUCTION

When my son, Matt was fifteen years old, I took him on his first fly-in fishing trip to a remote camp in Canada where we lived and fished with Ojibway Indians for one week. The fishing was great, but two days before we were scheduled to fly out, we witnessed a terrible accident. Two young Ojibways were splitting firewood when an ax head flew off the handle and struck one of the Indians in the head. Within seconds, the bleeding from a severe head wound became uncontrollable.

The Ojibways are superb woodsmen, but neither they nor I knew much about handling this kind of emergency. The camp did not have a first-aid kit and I carried only small bandages. We resorted to T-shirt bandages and masking tape to hold back most of the bleeding. When we could not stop the bleeding, we loaded the young Ojibway into a small boat and he was taken on a nine-hour trip to the closest reservation. I had doubts that he would survive.

About eight years ago, at a picnic, a friend suffered a heart attack. He dropped to the ground and his breathing stopped. Refusing to accept the fact that we'd lost a friend so quickly, some of us started CPR and mouth-to-mouth resuscitation. Our old friend started breathing again within a few minutes.

Fortunately, the young Ojibway Indian survived his accident as well.

As a hunter and fisherman, I have seen many less-serious accidents and illnesses in the outdoors, ranging from jellyfish and bee stings to fish hooks in the fingers and scratched eyeballs. I love the outdoors, but it can be dangerous if you're not prepared for the unexpected.

If you are sports-oriented, you want to "get away from the crowds and people," which is the way it should be, but never forget that you're also getting away from immediate medical help. You're on your own and your survival and the survival of others may well depend on how well you can handle an emergency.

The editors at *Outdoor Life* realized that this lack of basic medical training among hunters, fishermen, and campers is a contributing factor in the death or maiming of sportsmen and women every year from accidents and other emergencies that could probably have been treated or prevented, if treated immediately in the field. In the late 1980's, *Outdoor Life* announced a new monthly column, Sports Medicine. Its goal is simple: Teach *Outdoor Life* readers everything they need to know to stay physically fit in the outdoors.

About this time, we started to get a few articles from Paul G. Gill, Jr., M.D. His articles were always right on target and he spoke that special language of the hunter and fisherman. One of the first, as I recall, had to do with tree-stand injuries. Most doctors would probably have asked why a grown adult would be climbing into a tree in the first place, but not Paul. He is a deer hunter as well as a doctor. He knows that deer hunters occasionally fall out of tree stands.

Paul seemed too good to be true: a doctor who hunted, fished, camped, and hiked, and, perhaps most important to an editor, a doctor who could write well. When we discovered that Paul was a board-certified specialist and a member of the Wilderness Medical Society, *Outdoor Life* offered him the permanent position of Sports Medicine columnist.

Paul started his regular column for *Outdoor Life* back in 1988—and he has not disappointed me or his eight million readers with columns covering everything from fractures to toothaches to snakebites. Paul offers sound medical advice as well as tips on treatments you can find at your local drugstore. I expect Paul to bail us out of tight spots in the woods for many years to come.

Simon & Schuster's Pocket Guide to Wilderness Medicine is something you may need whenever you step outside. It is not optional gear: It's an essential piece of emergency equipment. At some point, if you spend enough time outdoors, this book may be the only thing between you and danger to your family or friends. I am not trying to scare anyone, but I have hunted and fished for enough years to know that everyone will eventually experience a health problem or an accident outdoors.

Finally, remember that the advice here comes from a doctor who knows the outdoors and its many potential dangers. This book is for all sportsmen and women looking for a place in the wilderness. It's for hunters who climb trees and sometimes fall out. It's for fishermen who cut their fingers and campers who get bellyaches. It's for all those outdoor people who want to learn how to take care of themselves and the friends who go with them.

VIN T. SPARANO,
Executive Editor, *Outdoor Life*

THE BASICS:
SHOCK, CPR, AND
THE ABCS

Travis MacKenzie was picking his way down the back side of Mount Mansfield in the Green Mountains of northern Vermont when he slipped on some loose shale and became airborne. He bounced and rolled several hundred feet down the mountain before his descent was abruptly arrested by a large and unyielding fir tree. Travis slammed into the tree, fracturing several ribs and rupturing his spleen. He lay on the ground, stunned, for several minutes before picking himself up and hobbling back onto the trail. He made it to a cabin halfway down the mountain, where he collapsed.

When hikers found him a couple of hours later, he was barely conscious. He lay shivering on a bunk, a low moan drifting from his bloodless lips with each fitful breath. His face was ashen and dappled with silvery beads of sweat, and his lusterless eyes were sunk into their sockets like pebbles dropped in the snow. A cold sweat glazed his skin, his fingers and nails were blue, and his pulse was a feeble thread. Travis MacKenzie was in shock.

ᖰ❧

Shock is war. Biologic blitzkrieg. When trauma or severe illness threatens the flow of oxygen- and nutrient-bearing blood to the body's tissues, the body responds with an all-out, banzai counterattack, formally known as shock.

As in all wars, the assault may take different forms: bleeding from open wounds, ruptured organs, or fractured bones (*"hemorrhagic shock"*); fluid loss from crush injuries, burns, heat exhaustion, severe diarrhea, snakebite, or uncontrolled diabetes; "pump failure" from massive heart attack; and vascular collapse secondary to insect sting, overwhelming infection, or spinal cord injury. Virtually any serious injury or illness can lead to shock.

Whatever the nature of the insult, the final result is the same: interruption of the flow of blood to the cells. Each cell in the body houses a miniature power plant where complex chemical reactions generate the energy that keeps our brain cells communicating with one another, the muscle fibers in our hearts contracting, and the rods and cones in our retinas reacting to light impulses. These reactions are fueled by a steady flow of oxygen and nutrients in the blood. When the flow of blood is cut off, the metabolic machinery grinds to a stop, just as an internal combustion engine sputters when it runs out of fuel.

When you think of shock, you think of gory wounds and blood. But internal bleeding can lead to shock, too. You can easily lose a couple of pints of blood from a fractured long bone, and you can bleed to death from a crushed pelvis or ruptured spleen or liver without ever seeing a drop of blood. Crush injuries are doubly dangerous because plasma, the noncellular component of blood, continues to leak from damaged blood vessels long after bleeding is controlled.

?~ THE BODY FIGHTS BACK

The body doesn't take blood loss lying down. The human machine is the end product of millions of years of evolution on a planet where dodging falling rocks and fighting saber-toothed tigers were all in a day's work. The response to blood loss starts when pressure sensors in the aorta and the carotid arteries in the neck detect a drop in blood pressure, and alert the vasomotor area of the brain, the shock "command post." The vasomotor area acts quickly to stabilize the circulation by stimulating the sympathetic nervous system (SNS), a special network of nerves supplying the heart and blood vessels. The SNS's response is three-pronged:

1. It stimulates the heart to beat harder and faster so that it delivers more oxygen and nutrients to tissues girding for combat.
2. It constricts the large veins throughout the body which serve as a reservoir for up to 50 percent of the blood in the circulatory tree. This is equivalent to an instant five-pint blood transfusion.
3. It clamps down on the small arteries in the muscles, intestines, skin, and kidneys, raising the blood pressure and diverting blood to the more vital brain and heart.

Meanwhile, the kidneys do their part by conserving salt and water, and the circulation receives a big boost in volume when fluid in the tissues ("extracellular fluid") passes into the blood vessels.

The body's compensatory mechanisms are very efficient. So efficient, in fact, that a young, otherwise healthy person can lose 25 to 30 percent of his blood volume (1,000 to 1,800 milliliters of blood, depending on his size) and show no signs of shock other than a rapid pulse and cool, moist skin. But if he loses even a few more milliliters of blood, he'll be on a slippery slope. Shock will become progressive and irreversible.

?❧ DIAGNOSIS

Trauma specialists talk about the "golden hour" in treating shock victims. If shock is not reversed within one hour, the patient will die, no matter what is done for him.

But shock has to be recognized before it can be treated. If your buddy falls out of a tree blind, how will you know if he is in shock? Ruptured spleens don't come with tags, and unless you have x-ray glasses, you can't see a fractured pelvis. But you don't need an MD after your name to recognize the classic signs of shock:

Mild Shock

The victim has lost up to a liter of blood, but his body is compensating well and his blood pressure remains normal. (*Beware:* estimating blood loss, especially your own, is like describing "the one that got away"—most people exaggerate.) He is alert, may complain of being cold and thirsty, and may feel weak and light-headed when he sits up. His skin is pale, cool, and damp, and his pulse is rapid, usually about 110 to 120 beats a minute.

Moderate Shock

Blood loss is substantial, 20 to 40 percent of his volume (1 to 2.5 liters), and the victim is prostrated. He is too weak to move under his own power, his speech is slurred, and he complains of thirst and shortness of breath. His skin is cold and clammy, his pulse is now very rapid and weak, and his urine output scant (less than 30 milliliters per hour).

Severe Shock

The victim has lost 40 percent or more of his

9

blood volume (2.5 liters or more), and blood flow to the heart and brain is now severely compromised. His breathing becomes shallow and rapid, his eyes become dull, his pupils dilate, and he becomes restless and agitated, then lethargic and comatose. Death is in the wings.

?❧ TREATMENT OF SHOCK

When shock is your foe, the battle has to be joined early. Once shock has progressed to the "severe" stage, the struggle is lost.

Treatment of the trauma victim starts with the ABCs: *a*irway, *b*reathing, and *c*irculation.

A. *Airway*. If he is unconscious, open his airway using the "jaw-thrust" technique: put a hand on each side of his face and lift the jaw up and forward *without tilting the head back* (unless you are sure that he does not have a neck injury).

B. *Breathing*. Check for breathing by listening to his mouth and chest and by observing his chest and abdomen. If you see chest and abdominal movement but don't hear breath sounds, check the airway again. If you still don't hear breath sounds, give two quick mouth-to-mouth breaths and go on to C.

C. *Circulation*. Put your index and middle fingers over the windpipe, and slide them down alongside the neck muscle and feel for a pulse. If there isn't one, start CPR (see later in this chapter).

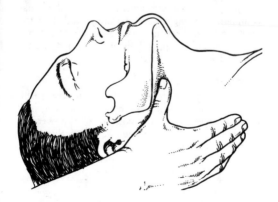

1. Opening the airway using the "jaw-thrust" technique.

Then do a quick head-to-toe survey for wounds and fractures, and splint any obvious fractures (see Chapter 4). Control bleeding by applying direct pressure to the wounds with any bulky, clean material—your shirt if nothing else is handy. Bright red blood spurting from a wound is arterial; oozing, dark blood is probably from a vein. Arterial bleeding, especially from the scalp, neck, groin, or shoulder, can be difficult to control and lead to rapid exsanguination. If firm pressure doesn't stop the bleeding after a few minutes, pack the wound with sterile gauze and cover it with a compression dressing. To control severe bleeding from a leg wound, push your fist into the abdomen directly above the navel and press firmly. This compresses the aorta against the spinal column and will control the flow of blood into the legs while you apply a bulky bandage. (This is the only "pressure point" you need to know about.) Tourniquets are dangerous. Don't use one unless you are willing to write off the limb to save the victim.

After you have controlled the bleeding, put the victim in the "shock position" with his legs flexed at the hips, knees straight, feet elevated 12 inches, and his head down. This promotes the return of venous blood to the heart and enhances the flow of arterial blood to the brain. (*Warning:* If the victim has chest injuries, this position may make it hard for him to breathe. In that case, keep him in a semisupine position.)

Conserve body heat by bundling him in blankets or an open sleeping bag, and offer him warm fluids by mouth if he is able to swallow.

Move him out of danger if you have to, but avoid rough handling. Check his vital signs every few minutes, including his pulse and breathing rate and pattern. Remember, restlessness and agitation may be signs of worsening shock.

Make arrangements for rapid medical evacuation. Time is of the essence!

Dealing with shock calls for courage, resourcefulness, and perseverance. General George Patton, "Old Blood and Guts," said it best: "A pint of sweat will save a gallon of blood."

ॐ CHOKING

When a diner chokes on a mouthful of filet mignon in a restaurant, it's called a "cafe coronary." When a hunter in a remote camp in Idaho (or anywhere else) chokes on a mouthful of food, it's called "sudden death"—unless his buddy knows the Heimlich maneuver and acts quickly.

Thousands of Americans choke to death on foreign bodies each year. The "foreign body" is usually a large, poorly chewed piece of meat. Many choking victims had been drinking alcohol or wear dentures. Both interfere with the normal swallowing reflex.

Airway obstruction is the most acute of all medical emergencies. The metabolic machinery of the brain cells is driven by oxygen. If the supply of oxygen is cut off for even a few seconds, it's "lights out." After three to five minutes without oxygen, the brain cells start to die, resulting in severe and irreversible brain damage.

Tragedy can be averted if you know what to do in an airway emergency and act quickly and deliberately. Your response to a choking emergency has to be reflexive and automatic, the way an experienced grouse hunter reacts to the sound of a bird taking wing. You have to know *beforehand* what you will do in every situation, and then do it without hesitation.

Remember the golden rule of medicine: "First do no harm." If the victim appears to be choking on a piece of food but is coughing and spluttering, *leave him alone!* His airway is only *partially* obstructed. Encourage him to cough hard, but resist the temptation to slap him on the back or perform the Heimlich maneuver. If he starts to make a high-pitched noise when he inhales, turns blue, and his coughs deteriorate into feeble little grunts, the obstruction is nearly complete. If he can't talk and is clutching his throat with his hands (the "universal airway distress signal"), the obstruction *is* complete. In either case, it's time for the Heimlich maneuver.

The Heimlich maneuver consists of a series of abdominal thrusts that elevate the diaphragm, the breathing muscle that separates the chest and abdominal cavities. Elevating the diaphragm causes a sudden rise in the pressure inside the chest cavity and an artificial cough that expels the foreign object. Here are the American Heart Association's recommendations on what to do when someone is choking:

1. *If the victim is standing or sitting and is conscious:* Stand behind him and wrap your arms around his waist. Make a fist with one hand, and place the thumb side of the fist against his abdomen, just above the navel. Grab your fist with your other

hand, and press it into his abdomen with a quick, upward thrust. Continue the thrusts until the airway is cleared or he loses consciousness. If he does lose consciousness, perform a "finger sweep": open his mouth by grasping the tongue and lower jaw and lifting (this pulls the tongue out of the back of the throat). Then insert the index finger of your other hand alongside the cheek to the base of the tongue. Hook the finger behind the object and remove it from the mouth. (Be careful not to push the object deeper into the throat!) Then, give a series of mouth-to-mouth breaths. If you can't ventilate the lungs, perform 6 to 10 abdominal thrusts, repeat the finger sweep and the mouth-to-mouth ventilations. Repeat the sequence of Heimlich maneuver, finger sweep, and mouth-to-mouth breathing until the airway is cleared.

2. *If the victim is lying on the ground unconscious:* Place him in a supine position, and kneel astride his thighs. Place the heel of one hand against his abdomen just above the navel, and put the other hand over the first. Press into the abdomen with a quick upward thrust. Repeat this supine Heimlich maneuver, the aforementioned finger sweep and ventilation sequence as necessary. (You can also use this technique with the conscious choking victim if your arms are too short to reach around his waist.)

3. *If the victim is very obese or pregnant and is conscious:* Stand behind him or her, and wrap your arms around his or her chest. Place the thumb side of your fist on the middle of the breastbone, grab your fist with the other hand, and perform a series of backward thrusts until the airway is cleared or he or she loses consciousness.

4. *If the victim is very obese or pregnant and is unconscious:* Place the victim on his or her back, kneel alongside him or her, and place the heel of your hand on the lower half of the breastbone. Place the other hand over the first, and perform a series of thrusts. As above, repeat Heimlich maneuvers, finger sweeps, and ventilations until the airway is cleared.

5. *If the choking victim is an infant:* This is the only situation in which back slaps are recommended. If you are sure that the child is choking on an object, and not suffering from a severe upper respiratory infection, position the child's head down so that his stomach is resting on your forearm while his arms and legs hang over on either side, and deliver four brisk blows between the shoulder blades with the heel of your hand. Then turn the infant face up,

position him on your thigh with his head down, and perform four chest thrusts, as described above.

6. *If you are alone and choking:* Perform the Heimlich maneuver on yourself. Make a fist with one hand, and place the thumb side on the abdomen just above the navel. Grab the fist with the other hand, and press inward and upward in a quick, sharp, thrusting motion. If this doesn't work, press your abdomen across any firm surface, such as a tree stump, rock, or outboard motor.

A *few caveats:* When doing abdominal or chest thrusts, be careful not to place the fist too close to the xiphoid process (a small piece of bone that projects down toward the abdomen from the breastbone) or on the lower margins of the rib cage. Fractures of the xiphoid or ribs can result in lacerations of the liver, spleen, or lungs. Also, abdominal thrusts can result in regurgitation of stomach contents, so try to position the victim so that his head is lower than the rest of the body. That way the stomach contents will drain out of the mouth and not obstruct the airway further.

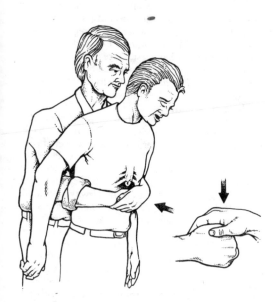

2. The Heimlich maneuver.

⁊☙ CARDIOPULMONARY RESUSCITATION

If your buddy keels over in the woods as a result of a cardiac arrest, he's going to The Happy Hunting Ground unless you can resuscitate him. The only way to become truly proficient at cardiopulmonary resuscitation (CPR) is by taking a course at your local hospital. When you've taken the course and become certified in CPR by the American Heart Association or American Red Cross, you'll be able to perform the ABCs. Here is a brief review of the techniques:

1. Airway: Establish that the victim is unresponsive, place him on his back on a firm, flat surface, and open his airway using the "head-tilt" technique. Place one hand under the victim's neck and the other on his forehead. Then, flex the neck and extend the head (see Figure 3).
2. Breathing: Kneel alongside the victim, and check to see if he is breathing by watching for movement of his chest and abdomen and listening for breath sounds with your ear against his chest. If he is not breathing, perform mouth-to-mouth breathing by pinching his nostrils, taking a deep breath, sealing your lips around his mouth, and giving him two full breaths.

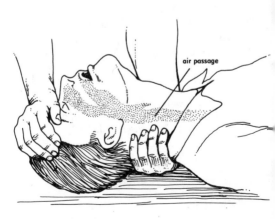

3. Opening the airway using the "head-tilt" technique.

3. Circulation: Check for pulses and, if absent, do chest compressions as follows:

a. Place the heel of one hand on the lower half of the breast bone, and place your other hand over the first.

b. Keeping your shoulders over his chest, and your elbows locked, compress the chest at a rate of 60 per minute, stopping every 15 compressions to open the airway and give two breaths. The breastbone should be depressed 1.5 to 2 inches with each compression.

c. *Caution!* Excessively forceful or misplaced compressions can cause fractures and injuries to internal organs. Don't let the heel of your hand slide down over the tip of the breastbone, and keep your fingers away from the chest.

If you *see* the victim collapse, quickly check for a pulse. If there is none, you may be able to restore his heartbeat with a sharp "thump" on the breastbone with your fist.

Continue CPR until

1. Breathing and pulses return.
2. The rescuers are exhausted.
3. The rescuers are in danger.
4. The victim fails to respond to prolonged resuscitation (how you define "prolonged" depends on the circumstances; prolonged CPR is more likely to be successful in hypothermia victims).
5. The rescuers are relieved by medical professionals.

CPR is not magic. There are situations when it shouldn't be attempted, including

1. A lethal injury (death is obvious).
2. A dangerous setting in which rescuers would be jeopardizing their own lives.
3. Chest compressions are impossible, e.g., the chest is frozen or crushed.
4. When any breathing or movement is evident.
5. The victim has clearly stated, in writing, that he doesn't want to be resuscitated.

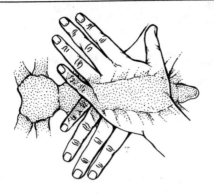

4. Proper hand position for chest compression.

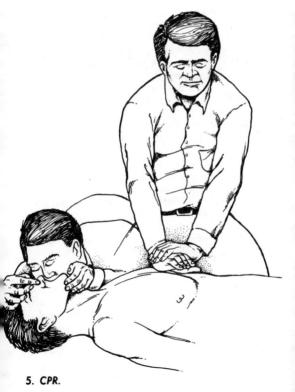

5. CPR.

2

SOFT-TISSUE INJURIES: SPRAINS, STRAINS, CUTS, AND BUMPS

It was the opening day of the spring turkey season, and Brian had been walking the ridges of New York's southern Adirondacks since daybreak. He stopped for a moment to rest and wipe the sweat from his brow. He shielded his eyes with his hands and looked up at the sun. The fiery ball was approaching its zenith. Another hour and he'd have to knock off for the day. He picked up his shotgun and headed down the steep, rock-strewn hillside, half-running in his haste to cover as much ground as possible before noon. Suddenly, his right foot went out from under him as he slipped on a rock. He felt an explosion of pain in his right ankle and went down in a heap, landing heavily on his right hip.

Brian saw stars for a few moments. His ankle felt as though it were the top of a ketchup bottle that Hulk Hogan was trying to unscrew. And his hip didn't feel so great either. He pulled up his pant leg, unlaced his boot and looked at his ankle. There was already a goose-egg-size swelling on the outside of it, but it didn't look broken. He ran his fingers over the bones. He couldn't feel any obvious fractures. If he could just make it back to camp, he'd soak it in some warm water with epsom salts and he'd be as good as new in the morning. There was no way he was not going hunting tomorrow, especially after being shut out today.

Brian limped back to camp, soaked his ankle in hot water, and slaked his thirst with a couple of cold beers. He would have been better off if he'd soaked his ankle in the cold beer and drunk the water—epsom salts and all. The beer took the edge off the pain; enough so that he spent most of the afternoon on his feet, hobbling around the camp making repairs. The next morning, his foot and ankle were so swollen they could have belonged to Big Foot. Brian

*couldn't get his boot on, and his hip was so sore he
couldn't raise his leg.*

ॐ

Through his ignorance of the basics of sprain care,
Brian converted a minor sprained ankle and contused hip into major, incapacitating injuries that ruined his spring turkey hunting. Treating these injuries
is simple if you keep a couple of elastic (Ace) bandages, a roll of tape, and instant ice packs in your
pack. But first, you have to understand the difference
between a sprain and a strain.

ॐ SPRAINS

A sprain is an injury to the ligaments around a
joint. (Knees, ankles, feet, toes, shoulders, elbows,
wrists, hands, and fingers can all be sprained. They
cannot be strained.) Ligaments are bands of tough,
thick fibrous tissue that hold joints together. When
sufficient stress is placed on a joint, the ligaments will
first stretch, and then tear as the stress is increased. In
a mild to moderate sprain, the ligament is stretched
and up to 75 percent of its fibers are torn. In a severe
sprain, all or nearly all of its fibers are torn.

Is It Broken?

Whenever you injure any joint, the most important question is: "Is it broken?" If you are 100 miles
from the nearest hospital, you are going to have to
make an educated guess. Here are some tip-offs to
fractures:

- Gently press on the bones around the injured joint.
  If there is a fracture, you may feel and hear the
  bone fragments rubbing together. This is called
  "crepitus."
- A fractured wrist or finger will look deformed, unless the fracture is hairline. If your wrist looks like
  an upside-down fork, it is broken.
- If the joint is dislocated, it will be obviously displaced.

Swelling alone is not a reliable guide to the severity of an injury. Mild sprains may look much worse
than many fractures. You can usually walk, although
with pain, on a sprained ankle or foot. If the thin
bone on the outside of the ankle (the fibula) is broken, you may still be able to walk on that leg because
the fibula is not a weight-bearing bone. The majority
of ankle and foot fractures, though, are too painful

to walk on. If your wrist is broken, your grip will be weak. You won't be able to hold a cup of coffee in that hand.

Treatment

RICE is the key to treating sprains. Not the kind they throw at weddings. RICE is the acronym for *r*est, *i*ce, *c*ompression, and *e*levation. The objectives in the initial treatment of sprains are (1) to limit swelling and bleeding and (2) to relieve pain. Swelling increases pain and prolongs healing. You've got to move fast to prevent it. A sprained ankle will balloon up right in front of your eyes. Reducing swelling after it has already happened is like trying to put toothpaste back into the tube. And the more you move the injured joint, the more it's going to bleed. So rest it.

Ice does two things: it slows bleeding from torn vessels, limiting swelling, and it deadens the sensory nerves in the injured area. There's no better painkiller for a sprain than a bag of ice (a cold mountain stream will do in a pinch). But watch for frostbite: don't apply the ice directly to the skin. Lay a towel over the injured joint and rest the bag on the towel.

An elastic bandage wrapped around a sprained ankle or wrist provides compression that also prevents bleeding and swelling. Apply the ice over the bandage for 30 minutes. Then, remove the ice and bandage to allow blood to flow into the injured area. After 15 minutes, reapply the elastic bandage and ice bag. You can repeat this cycle as many times as you like during the first 24 to 48 hours. Just be sure that the bandage isn't wrapped too tightly. If your toes or fingers start to hurt, tingle, or turn white or blue, remove the bandage immediately.

Keep the injured extremity elevated above heart level. (For example, if you sprain your ankle, put a pillow or rolled-up jacket under it while you're lying down.) This reduces swelling by promoting drainage of blood and fluids from the injury.

If there are still pain and swelling after 48 hours of RICE, substitute warm soaks or compresses for ice. Continue to elevate the part as much as possible, and keep it wrapped in a pressure dressing or splint when it's not soaking.

When the pain subsides, start to use the extremity. But be careful! Take those first steps as though you were walking on eggshells. If you overdo it, you will turn your healing sprain into a fresh sprain, and it may never heal properly. You'll end up with permanently stretched, loose ligaments and an unstable joint ("chronic sprain"). When you can walk without pain, or use the wrist, hand, or shoulder comfortably, put away the elastic bandage and head back into the field. But be aware that it takes up to six months for torn ligaments to regain maximum strength.

Wrist injuries should be splinted as follows: Put a rolled-up pair of socks in the palm of the hand and rest the wrist and hand on a 10-inch-long piece of cardboard or wooden slat. Then wrap an elastic bandage around the hand from the knuckles to about 6 inches above the wrist. This is a "cock-up" splint. It keeps the wrist bent back in a natural, comfortable position, and will prevent the hand from getting stiff. This is also the best way to immobilize a sprained or badly bruised hand. (A word of caution about "sprained" wrists: There is no way that anyone, even a doctor, can tell if a wrist is fractured without x-rays. As soon as you get home, have your doctor look at it. An untreated wrist fracture can result in permanent loss of function of the hand and chronic pain and disability.)

Use the buddy system for sprained fingers and toes. Tape the injured digit to its partner. Then ice and elevate it.

?• STRAINS

Strains are muscle injuries. Muscles can be "pulled," meaning that the muscle contracts so forcefully during a sudden movement that it either rips the tendon out of the bone or the muscle rips away from the tendon. Or the muscle itself can tear. Strains are every bit as painful as sprains, and take about as long to heal. Not surprisingly, the treatment is almost the same: RICE for 24 to 72 hours, followed by range-of-motion exercises in warm water (hydrotherapy) three times a day. The warm water relaxes the muscle and promotes circulation of nutrient-carrying blood to the healing tissues. Continue hydrotherapy until you have regained full, pain-free use of the muscle.

?• CONTUSIONS

Brian developed a big, tender, black and blue discoloration on his hip. A deep bruise like this is called a *contusion*. The force of Brian's weight landing on his hip resulted in a crush injury to the skin and underlying muscle and bone. Blood vessels in the skin and muscle ruptured, causing black and blue marks ("ecchymoses") on the skin and a pool of blood in the muscle called a "hematoma." Contusions and hematomas are treated in the same way as strains, and take about 4 to 5 days to heal. Large contusions can be quite painful, and may mask serious underlying injury. A hard blow to the back can cause a contused kidney, usually manifested as blood in the urine. A severe blow to the chest can cause a contused lung, which will cause shortness of breath and coughing up blood.

⁊ SUBUNGUAL HEMATOMAS

When you drop a rock on the end of your finger, the nail bed (the tissue under the nail) bleeds into the confined space under the nail. As the pressure builds up under the nail, the nail turns blue and the pain becomes exquisite. The simplest remedy is to drain the hematoma with a hot paper clip. Or you can drill a hole in the nail with a knife or needle point. (First make certain that the end of the finger isn't fractured: push down against the tip—if it is not particularly tender, it is probably not fractured.)

⁊ OPEN WOUNDS

Open wounds can be produced by sharp, blunt, cutting, or crushing objects, and are characterized by a break in the body's first line of defense against infection, the skin. Regardless of their size, shape or location, the objectives in treating an open wound in the wilderness are the same:

1. Prevent shock by controlling bleeding (see Chapter 1).
2. Prevent infection by thorough cleaning of the wound.
3. Promote healing by application of sterile dressings and splinting.

Control Bleeding

Most bleeding can be controlled with firm pressure over the wound or direct pressure with your fingertips over the bleeding vessels (see Chapter 1).

Cleaning the Wound

After you've stopped the bleeding, the next step is to examine the wound. First wash your hands; then check to see how deep the wound is, and whether there is any damage to deep structures such as bones, nerves, tendons, and blood vessels. Remove pebbles, vegetable matter, and other foreign objects by hand, and then cleanse the wound with the cleanest water available, which in most cases will be your drinking water. Stream water is fine once it has been disinfected (see Chapter 16). Add a little 10 percent povidone-iodine solution to make a 1 percent solution, and irrigate the wound liberally, taking pains to wash out grit, soil, and vegetable matter. Use a sterile gauze pad to gently wipe dirt out of the wound. (Scrubbing further traumatizes the tissues, increasing bleeding and the risk of infection.)

The best way to dislodge small dirt particles from the wound is by injecting the solution under pressure with a syringe. Direct the stream into the depths of the wound, under skin flaps, and at any particles that seem to be adherent to the wound. When you're done irrigating the wound, make a final inspection and remove any debris that may be left in the wound.

Closing the Wound

Many wounds are best left "open" in a wilderness setting. No matter how meticulous you are in cleansing the wound, it is virtually impossible to remove all contaminants from a wound when your operating theater is a clearing in the forest and the operating table is a bed of pine needles. Bacteria thrive on the blood and necrotic debris that accumulate in the depths of a contaminated wound. Closing such a wound is a recipe for wound infection. If you leave the wound open, pus can drain freely and won't accumulate to form an abscess. But each wound has to be treated based on its specific characteristics, including location, depth, contamination, and injury to deep structures.

It is generally safe to close facial and scalp lacerations. They rarely become infected, thanks to the rich blood supply to the head. Large scalp wounds usually have to be closed to control bleeding. The simplest way to do this is to tie clumps of hair across the wound until the bleeding stops (hair doesn't hold a knot well, so use double square knots). Most facial lacerations can be closed nicely with micropore tape (see Chapter 23). Apply a little tincture of benzoin to the skin on either side of the wound to make the tape stick better (be careful not to get any in the wound itself—it stings!). Then dab a little triple antibiotic ointment on the wound (it doesn't prevent infection, but it does stimulate healing). When the benzoin has dried, apply several tapes across the wound. The best technique is to first anchor one end of the tape to a wound edge and then pull that edge up snug to the opposite edge, making sure that the wound edges are even. If kept dry, these micropore tapes will stay in place until the wound has healed, usually 5 to 7 days.

Larger lacerations can be closed very nicely with staples. 3M Corporation makes a disposable five-staple device called the "Precise Five-Shot." It comes with a device for removing the staples (after 5 days for facial lacerations, 7 days for scalp lacerations, 10 days for upper extremity lacerations, and 14 days for lower extremity lacerations.)

Lacerations on the trunk and extremities should be cleaned as well as possible, skin edges stapled together, coated with antibiotic ointment, and covered with a sterile dressing in layers. The first layer should be a sterile, nonabsorbent dressing, such as Vaseline gauze (Adaptic, Johnson & Johnson). This is an open-mesh fabric impregnated with a petroleum emulsion that allows blood and other fluids to seep through the mesh. It doesn't stick to the wound, so dressing changes aren't painful. The next layer should be absorbent sterile pads (Nu Gauze, Johnson & Johnson), followed by a large surgical dressing (Surgipad, Johnson & Johnson) if the laceration is large and compression is needed to control bleeding. The dressings can then be taped in place or wrapped with roller gauze. If you don't have staples on hand, use steri-strips, or simply bandage the wound after dressing.

If the wound is particularly dirty, wet-to-dry dressings may be the best approach. Apply wet sterile gauze pads directly to the wound, and change them twice a day. When the dressing is dry, you remove it along with crust and debris. This is an effective way to control infection in any wound. (An antibiotic effective against staph bacteria, such as Duricef, should be started if the wound turns red and tender, drains pus, or if the victim develops a fever.)

Skin Avulsions and Flaps

When a knife or other sharp object strikes the skin at a shallow angle, it often tears off a hunk of skin. This is called an *avulsion*. Avulsions come in two forms: partial-thickness, in which just the top layers of the skin are lost, and full-thickness, in which all of the skin and possibly some of the underlying tissue is lost. Fingertips are frequently avulsed when the victim is slicing a loaf of bread or a slab of meat. A glancing blow from an axe may avulse a piece of skin from the leg.

Avulsions are treated in virtually the same way as lacerations, except no attempt should be made to close an avulsion. Since skin is missing, the wound has to heal from the bottom out. All fingertip avulsions heal, providing bone isn't exposed. Exposed bone needs to be covered with a skin graft. And any avulsion larger than a half-dollar will generally require skin grafting.

A flap is basically an avulsion in which the skin and underlying fatty tissue are intact on one side. A flap will often survive if its blood supply is good. A pale flap has no blood supply, and can be expected to gradually turn black and fall off. But it can still serve as a "biologic dressing" while the wound heals from beneath. Flaps should be gently cleaned with antiseptic solution and then bandaged. If the wound turns red and starts to drain pus, infection has set in. The flap can be lifted off to promote drainage, and wet-to-dry dressings applied.

?❧ PUNCTURE WOUNDS

Puncture wounds can be treacherous. The wound may not look like much, but that rusty nail, thorn, or wood splinter may have driven bacteria and dirt deep into the tissues. It also may have punctured a blood vessel, nerve, tendon, or joint lining. These are "tetanus-prone" wounds that must be thoroughly irrigated with antiseptic solution, preferably with a high-pressure syringe. Then you can apply antibiotic ointment and a light dressing. (Make sure that your tetanus immunization is up to date before you leave home.)

How to Remove a Fish Hook

There is no easy way to remove a fish hook embedded in your arm, leg, or ear. But there is a sure way. Clean the skin around the wound, and then numb the area by applying an ice cube (if you have one) directly to the skin over the point of the hook. Then, grab hold of the shank of the hook with a pair of needle-nose pliers and quickly pull the point of the hook through the skin. Snip off the barb, and back the hook out. Then soak the wound in antiseptic solution for a few minutes, and apply some antibiotic ointment and a bandage strip.

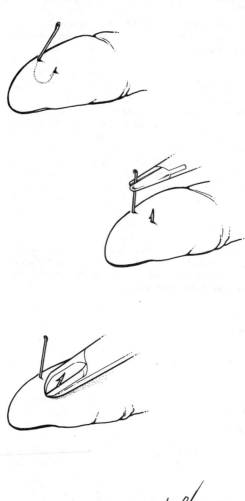

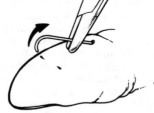

6. *How to remove a fish hook.*

How to Remove Splinters

Splinters are always harder to remove than you think. And your best shot at removing a splinter is your first. The more you poke at it, the more fragmented it becomes, the farther you push it into the wound, and the less cooperative is the victim. So sit him and yourself down, pull up a good light, and get out your finest tweezers. Before you start, press on the skin around the entrance wound, and get a feel for the orientation of the splinter under the skin. Put your finger against the point of the splinter that is embedded in the skin, and push it toward the entrance wound. Then, get a good hold of the exposed portion of the thorn or splinter with your tweezers, and pull in the opposite direction to that in which it entered the skin. After you get the splinter out, wash the wound with antiseptic solution, and apply antibiotic ointment and a dressing.

Large impaled objects should be left in place, especially if they are in the eye, neck, chest, or abdomen. In the old Westerns, they were always in a big hurry to pull the arrow out of the cavalryman's back. In real life, that's a big no-no. That arrow, stake, or what-have-you may be the only thing preventing catastrophic bleeding from a perforated blood vessel. Instead, stabilize the object by wrapping it in a bulky bandage, then evacuate the victim to a hospital.

?❧ ABRASIONS

An abrasion is what you get when you skin your knee or elbow, or scrape the superficial layer of skin over any bony prominence, such as the front of the leg, knuckles, or chin. Dirt may be ground into these wounds, so you need to spend some time washing them, using either a mild soap or an antiseptic solution. Small abrasions can be covered with a transparent dressing, such as Bioclusive (Johnson & Johnson) or Tegaderm adhesive dressings (3M). These are waterproof dressings that "breathe." They keep water out but allow oxygen to penetrate to the healing tissues, and they can be left on for several days. Larger abrasions should be bandaged the same way as a laceration—with antibiotic ointment, a nonabsorbent dressing, and a few layers of absorbent gauze for compression. The dressing should be changed daily until a firm scab forms (resist the temptation to pick off the scab—it's a natural dressing).

3

BURNS

It was cold that morning out on the bay. A bitter cold that bit straight through to the bone. The kind that quickly numbs you, taking your mind off the burning pain in your fingers, nose and ears, slowing the reflexes and dulling thought.

There weren't many birds moving. The air was still, and although Jim had seen a mallard and a black duck, he hadn't been able to call them in. It was almost as though the waterfowl on the bay knew that this was the last day of hunting season. Jim didn't know how much longer he was going to want to sit out here, slowly freezing to death in a duck boat. He stretched his legs, in the process kicking the small gasoline heater that he had thrown in the boat the night before. He looked down at it for a second, regarding it as Pandora might have scrutinized her infamous box. He knew he shouldn't have brought it. He could think of a dozen good reasons not to use it in the duck boat. He quickly shoved aside common sense, pulled out a book of matches, and lit the wick. Soon the top of the heater was aglow and sending up shimmering waves of warm air. He pushed it down by his feet and turned his attention back to waterfowl.

A pair of mallards came into view, high in the eastern sky. Jim started calling. They flew by, apparently uninterested, but then veered around to take another look. He called frantically, and then dropped the call and slowly picked up his 12-gauge side-by-side as they approached the pattern of decoys from the leeward side. They were coming in, wings spread in a classic pose as they slowed and prepared to glide into the water alongside their plastic mates. Jim nudged the safety forward, sat bolt upright, and fired, knocking down two ducks and knocking over one gasoline heater in the bottom of his duck boat.

Seconds later, the boat was engulfed in flames. Encumbered by his hip boots and bulky clothing, Jim struggled out of the inferno and then ran down the shore as fast as he could in the oozing, clinging, black mud. He didn't want to be around when the flames reached the outboard motor fuel tank. It exploded seconds later with a tremendous roar and a blast of heat that he could feel twenty yards away. He took a quick look at the disintegrating hulk of his duck boat and then waded out into the cold water of the bay, where he ripped off his smoldering gloves and thrust his burned hands into the frigid water. After the pain in his hands eased, he splashed water onto his stinging cheeks and forehead.

?•

Jim was a lucky guy. A fellow hunter took him to a hospital, where the doctor told him he had escaped with partial-thickness burns of his hands and face. While he lay on a stretcher with cool bandages draped across his face and each hand immersed in a basin of cold water, the doctor explained that these burns involved only the top layers of the skin, and that they would heal with little scarring. Full-thickness burns would have destroyed all layers of the skin and would have necessitated hospitalization and skin grafting.

Jim's story illustrates three points about burns. They are nearly always preventable. They nearly always happen at an inconvenient time. And they *usually* cause more pain than permanent injury.

Whether the result of fire, chemicals, electricity, or exposure to hot water or steam, burn injuries are entirely preventable, *especially* in the field. If your cabin or duck boat catches fire, chances are it's due to some mistake on your part rather than arson.

?• HOW TO APPROACH BURNS

Presumably, you put out the fire and removed the smoldering clothing from the burn victim before you picked up this book. The next step is to evaluate the severity of the burn. This is determined by the depth, size, and location of the burn and the age of the victim.

Grading Burns

Partial-thickness burns are red and painful, and may have large blisters. If they are red and painful without blisters, they are first-degree burns. Blisters indicate that they are second-degree burns. With these burns, the hair follicles and nerve endings are undamaged, and sensation is preserved. If infection is kept at bay, these burns will heal.

Full-thickness (third-degree) burns have a charred, leathery or waxy appearance. Ironically, since the skin is destroyed, so are its nerve endings, and full-thickness burns are virtually painless. Full-thickness burns larger than a silver dollar usually require skin grafting.

The size of the burn is expressed in terms of the percentage of body surface burned. The easiest way to do this is to use the "rule of nines." The head is considered to be 9 percent, the front and back of the torso each 18 percent, each upper extremity 9 percent, each lower extremity 18 percent, and the genitals 1 percent of the body surface area.

Partial-thickness burns involving less than 10 percent of the body can be considered *minor* and treated with the materials on hand in your medical kit. Apply cool compresses for a few minutes to give immediate relief of pain. Then, gently clean the burn with disinfected water and a mild soap or antiseptic solution, using a cotton ball to remove dirt and debris. An intact blister is sterile and should be left alone. Once it is opened, it is vulnerable to infection. All burns with blisters, open or closed, should be covered with a thin (⅛-inch) layer of triple antibiotic or silver sulfadiazine (Silvadene) cream and covered with a fine-mesh roll gauze bandage and then bulkier dry (Kling) gauze bandage. Fingers and toes are bandaged individually. The dressing should be carefully loosened with warm water and removed daily, the burn washed with mild soap (Dial or Ivory), and then re-dressed. By changing the dressings daily, whatever pus and necrotic debris have accumulated in the preceding 24 hours are removed, and the wound is kept clean. *A partial-thickness burn will heal if it doesn't become infected,* usually within 7 to 10 days. Burns are tetanus-prone wounds, so make sure your tetanus booster is up to date. Ibuprofen, up to 2,400 mg a day, or Tylenol No. 3, one or two every 4 hours, will take the edge off the pain of an extensive burn.

The following types of burns are to be considered *major burns:* second-degree burns covering more than 10 percent or third-degree burns over more than 5 percent of the body; most burns involving the face, eyes, ears, hands, feet, and genitals; circumferential burns; burns associated with fractures and other significant trauma; and less severe burns in anyone less than 5 or greater than 60 years of age. These people should be rapidly stabilized and evacuated to a hospital. When the body is denuded of a significant amount of its covering, shock from fluid loss and overwhelming infection is inevitable unless fluid is replaced and the burns covered with sterile dressings. While awaiting medical evacuation, keep the extremities elevated to promote drainage, and encourage the burn victim to take fluids by mouth if he is alert and in no respiratory distress.

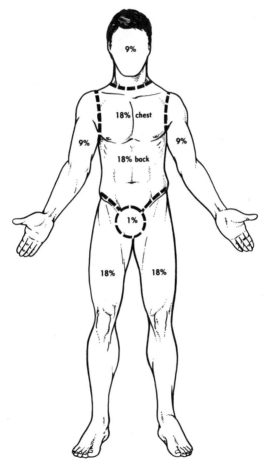

7. The "rule of nines."

Space Heaters

Jim had no business using the gasoline heater in the small confines of a duck boat. Such heaters are intended for use only in well-ventilated areas away from combustibles. Kerosene heaters used to heat cabins or tents are very economical and efficient. They are also very dangerous. They can start a conflagration if knocked over (although newer models have automatic fuel shut-off features), and emit dangerous concentrations of toxic gases. They should be operated only in well-ventilated structures, and the fuel supply should be kept outside.

Chemical Burns

There is a long list of caustic chemicals which can cause serious burns, but the sportsman in the field is not likely to come into contact with any of these except the sulfuric acid in his car or boat battery—and then only if he causes the battery to explode through improper use of jumper cables. (Always first connect one end of the red cable to the positive terminal of the good battery, the other end to the positive terminal of the dead battery. Then connect one end of the black cable to the negative terminal of the good battery, and the other end to the *engine block* of the vehicle with the dead battery.) Skin that has come in contact with the 28 percent solution of sulfuric acid in 12-volt batteries has a red appearance, signifying first-degree burns. When the eyes are exposed to the acid they become very red and teary and the lids swell. Treatment of battery burns consists, first of all, of removing all wet clothing and then thorough washing of all burned areas with voluminous amounts of water. A thin layer of Silvadene is soothing and will help prevent infection. If the eyes are burned, they should be washed under running water for at least 15 minutes. Flip over the lids and thoroughly irrigate the recess where the lid meets the eyeball. Then patch the eye and hurry to the nearest hospital. Time is of the essence if permanent scarring of the cornea is to be averted.

Gasoline and kerosene can cause painful burns when spilled on exposed skin. Treatment is the same as for sulfuric acid burns.

A pot of boiling water can be knocked off a campfire or portable stove just as easily as off the kitchen stove back home. The result is the same, of course: partial-thickness burns with large blisters or full-thickness burns. Treat them the same as any other thermal burn.

Electrical Burns

Portable gas-powered generators have become popular among sportsmen hunting or fishing in remote areas. These units can really turn on the juice (120 volts, the same as house voltage), and must be handled with great respect. So-called flash burns are partial-thickness burns that result from exposure to an electrical flash or explosion. They are treated just like any other partial-thickness burn. "Arc burns," which result when the electrical current directly contacts the skin, are horses of another color. They are far more serious and result from electrical current passing through the body from a point of entry to a point of exit. In the low-voltage arc burns that usually result from these generators, current accumulates at the points of entrance and exit, and these two areas are more badly burned than underlying tissues. If entrance and exit wounds are on either side of the chest or on the hands, the current may have taken a path through the heart, possibly injuring it. And it may have caused serious thermal injury to blood vessels, nerves, bones, and other structures in its path. Since arc burns are almost always full-thickness, they must be treated at the nearest hospital. The best way to avoid electrical burns from these generators is to become thoroughly familiar with their operation before leaving home. Never try to hook them up in the dark.

Friction Burns

Friction or "rope" burns can range from mild superficial abrasions to deep thermal burns and shredding of the skin of the palms of the hands or other unprotected body parts. They are treated in the same manner as other burns. You should always pack a pair of rawhide work gloves.

FRACTURES AND DISLOCATIONS

Rick held his breath as he lined up the big elk in his cross hairs. He held on the area right behind its shoulder, and slowly squeezed the trigger. Too slowly. The elk moved just as he fired. The wounded bull bounded into a stand of lodgepole pines on the far side of the ravine. Rick shouldered his rifle and headed down the slope at a run, slipping and sliding on the rock-strewn ground. Halfway down he stumbled over a log and his feet went out from under him. He reached up and grabbed an overhanging branch to break his fall, and yelled out in anguish as his shoulder popped out of joint like a cork out of a bottle.

Mac, Rick's partner, had heard the shot and was at his side in seconds. Rick was lying on his back moaning, his left arm sticking out from his side at an odd angle. Mac loosened Rick's jacket and shirt, and ran his hand over Rick's shoulder. It was dislocated. His eyes wandered down to Rick's arm and hand. They were cold and blue. He quickly felt his wrist for a pulse. There was none.

ॐ

Can you imagine trying to pack out an elk with a dislocated shoulder? You'd feel like a one-armed paperhanger. Your partner could pop it back in for you, if he knew how. Otherwise, you'd be lucky to get *yourself* out. Fractures and dislocations are big-time injuries. They should ideally be treated by a physician. But if you're hunting elk in Wyoming or fishing for golden trout in some remote mountain lake in Idaho, you won't want to wait several hours to be helicoptered to some distant hospital before getting your hip put back in socket. And if your dislocated shoulder is pressing on nerves and blood vessels, causing your arm to turn blue, you need help fast.

৵ EVALUATING THE INJURY

The first step in treating a fracture in the wild is to check the circulation, motor function, and sensation (CMS) of the limb beyond the injured area. After all, a fracture is nothing more than a soft-tissue injury complicated by a broken bone. How you handle an injured extremity depends primarily on the results of this initial exam. If you find a loss of motor power, sensation, or circulation in the limb, that means that the bone ends are pressing on the vessels or nerves at the fracture site, and gangrene or permanent paralysis could result if you don't remedy the situation. Here's how you do a CMS exam:

Circulation: Gently remove the boot and sock if the lower extremity is injured, or glove or mitten if the upper, and feel for pulses. Feel at the wrist on the thumb side, and right behind the inner knob at the ankle, or on the top of the foot between the first and second metatarsals (long bones). Then check the warmth and color of the fingers and toes. They should be pink. If they are blue or pale and cold, the circulation is impaired.

Motion: Ask the victim to wiggle his fingers or toes and to flex and extend his wrist or ankle.

Sensation: Check for perception of light touch, pressure, and pinprick.

The next step is to make an educated guess as to whether you *are* dealing with a fracture or just a bad sprain, meaning that the bones are intact but the ligaments around the joint are torn. (By the way, a "fractured" bone is the same as a "broken" bone.) A sprained ankle can swell to the size of a grapefruit in a matter of minutes. And a badly bruised shoulder or thigh can look for all the world as though it's broken. But you don't need a portable x-ray machine to diagnose a fracture. Press gently on the bone. If it's broken you'll feel a crunchy sensation (crepitus) as the bone ends rub together (and you'll elicit some colorful language from the victim). Compare the injured limb with its opposite. Do they look the same? Can the victim move the limb through a full range of motion? If so, it's probably not fractured.

Next, check the skin over the fracture. If bone is protruding from the skin, you are looking at an open, or "compound," fracture. Put the cleanest possible dressing on the wound before you do anything else. Then splint the limb, and give the victim Duricef, 1 gram immediately and 500 mg every 12 hours. There is a danger of bone infection (osteomyelitis) and gangrene in any open fracture, and these people have to be evacuated to a hospital as quickly as possible.

If the bones are bent at an odd angle, you need to bring them back into alignment. Here is why it's important to set, or "reduce," an obvious fracture:

1. To relieve the pressure of bone ends pressing on nerves and blood vessels.
2. To stop bleeding at the fracture site.
3. To prevent a closed fracture from becoming an open fracture.
4. To relieve pain.
5. So that you can apply a splint to the limb.

After stabilizing the fracture, a decision will have to be made regarding evacuation. Some fractures can be definitively treated in the field. Others will be angulated and require reduction under anesthesia. Reduction of uncomplicated fractures can be put off for up to seven days without jeopardizing the final result; but any open fracture or fracture associated with significant blood loss, spinal cord injury, or nerve or circulatory impairment must be evaluated quickly.

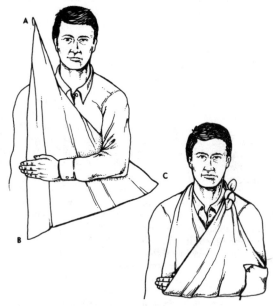

8. Making a sling. A goes behind neck then ties to B; fold C over and pin.

?❤ SPLINTS AND SLINGS

You can't apply a cast, obviously, but you *can* effectively immobilize most fractures with splints made from rope, brush and tree branches, metal pack frames, rifles, shotgun barrels, arrows, pack straps, sleeping pads, newspapers, and maps. On a long trek, you'd be smart to bring along a selection of wire, pneumatic or padded aluminum splints. Splinting the fracture in the functional position will decrease bleeding and damage to soft tissues, prevent stiffness, and make the victim more comfortable. The splint should immobilize the joints above and below the fracture. It should provide some compression, but not so much that it cuts off the circulation. Loosen any compressive bandages or wraps every two hours to check CMS, and don't forget the RICE: *r*est, *i*ce, *c*ompression, and *e*levation.

?❤ FRACTURES OF THE UPPER EXTREMITY

Collarbone

Fractures of the collarbone are usually obvious. After a fall onto the shoulder, you'll have swelling and crepitus over the middle of the collarbone and pain on upward movement of the arm. The classic treatment for these fractures is a figure-of-eight splint. Make a long splint out of cloth. Stand behind the victim and pass the ends over his shoulders, then under the armpits (which must be well-padded), and tie them in the back. Make sure the splint is snug, but not too tight. (You should just be able to insert two fingers under the splint where it passes over a shoulder blade.) The idea is to draw the shoulders back to minimize overlapping of the bone ends. Wear a sling for a few days to take the weight off of the arm on the side of the fracture.

Shoulder

A hard fall on the side or back of the shoulder can crack the upper arm bone (humerus) near the shoulder. There will be marked swelling and inability to use the arm. A fractured shoulder blade is just one of the injuries you can get when a tree jumps out in front of you while you are cross-country skiing. A violent impact against the shoulder blade will crack it like an eggshell. Both of these fractures do well in a sling and swathe. You can make a sling out of a triangular bandage, a shirt, or a large piece of cloth.

Rest the injured arm in the sling, keeping the hand accessible so that you can check the pulse periodically, and strap it against the chest with an elastic bandage or any material that you can wrap around the arm and chest. This will hold the arm in a comfortable position.

Upper Arm

Fractures of the mid-upper arm are problematic. These are unstable fractures, and muscle forces cause the fracture to bow forward. A common complication of mid-humerus fractures is "wristdrop," inability to extend the wrist or fingers due to pressure on the nerve that supplies the wrist and finger extensor muscles. Immobilize these fractures by firmly applying wood slats or similar materials to both the inner and outer aspects of the upper arm and securing them with an elastic bandage. Then put the arm in a sling and swathe. If there is a wristdrop, splint it in a position of function with a "cock-up splint" (see later).

Elbow

The elbow doesn't have much padding. If you slip on a rock and land on your elbow, it's not the rock that's going to crack. Immobilize fractures of the elbow in a sling with the elbow bent at roughly a right angle.

Forearm

Fractures of both bones in the forearm are unstable, and should be firmly splinted and then put in a sling. If the forearm is badly deformed and CMS is impaired, take hold of the arm by the wrist and apply steady, gentle traction. When the arm looks straight, splint it and put the arm in a sling. Sure, it'll hurt a little. But reducing the fracture will do wonders for the circulation to the arm and hand, and your buddy will be much more comfortable when his fractured wing is splinted and resting in a sling. Be sure to check the CMS of the fingers at regular intervals after you reduce the fracture. Loosen the splint if the pulse is weak, if there is any loss of motion or sensation in the fingers, or if they turn blue or white.

Wrist

If, after a fall on the outstretched hand, the wrist looks like an upside-down fork, it's fractured. But one of the small bones could be fractured and not produce a deformity. If there is any question of a fracture, make a "cock-up" splint: Put a rolled-up pair of socks in the palm of the hand and rest the wrist and hand on a 10-inch-long piece of cardboard or wooden slat. Then wrap an elastic bandage around the hand from the knuckles to about 6 inches above the wrist. This will keep the wrist and hand in a natural, comfortable position, and prevent it from getting stiff. (This is also a good way to splint a sprained or badly contused hand.) If you can't find a pulse at the wrist, or the fingers are cold and blue, you may be dealing with a fracture-dislocation. Reduce it by grasping the victim's hand in yours, handshake fashion, and pull straight out until the deformity is corrected. Check the circulation, and then splint as above.

Hand

Fractures of the long bones of the hand are usually stable and require nothing more than an elastic bandage or a cock-up splint. Reduce angulated fractures of the fingers by pulling straight out on the injured digit. Splint the finger with an aluminum splint or by taping it to the adjoining finger ("buddy splint"). Crushed fingertips should be thoroughly cleaned, dressed, and then protected with a short splint applied to the last third of the finger.

?❧ FRACTURES OF THE SPINE AND LOWER EXTREMITY

Back

Most back injuries are due to twisting, bending, or lifting movements that injure the muscles, ligaments, and discs of the lower (lumbar) spine. These generally respond to a day or two of bed rest, along with warm compresses and analgesics.

Falling off a cliff never hurt anyone. It's those hard landings that will get you every time. Rapid deceleration produces tremendous compression forces which can crush the vertebral bodies, usually in the midback area. A severe injury will result in fracture-dislocation of the spine. In a situation like this, you have to assume that the spinal cord is injured until you find evidence to the contrary (see Chapter 5). If the victim has to be moved, logroll him to avoid further injury to the spinal cord. Then do a quick neurologic exam: Check his grasp strength, then ask him to wiggle his toes and bend his knees and hips. Check to see whether he can feel light touch, pressure, and pinprick over the arms, legs, and trunk. If his motor strength and sensation are normal, roll him onto one side and check for fractures by gently thumping over the entire spinal column. If you find a tender area, you can assume that there is a compression fracture at that level. Gently roll him back onto his back, check for other injuries, and arrange for medical evacuation. If the neurologic exam is normal, and you don't find any tender areas in the spine, you can assume that there is no serious spinal injury and tend to his other injuries.

Pelvis, Hip, and Thigh

Fractures of the hip, pelvis, and thighbone (femur) are potential killers. You can easily lose a quart of blood from one of these fractures. Pelvic fractures are frequently multiple and can result in massive blood loss, shock, and tears in the bladder. Such injuries in the wilderness will challenge your resourcefulness and will. Here is how you handle them: If a fractured pelvis or hip is suspected and weight bearing is painful, place the victim in a supine position. If he complains of pain in the groin, and the leg appears shorter than the other and is rotated outward, he probably has a fracture of the hip. Splint the fracture by strapping the legs together. Make a litter or sled, put him on it, and head for home. (A roll under the knees will make him a little more comfortable during the trip.) Stop periodically and check for signs of shock: pale, cool, wet skin, rapid, thready pulse, and agitation.

Fractures of the shaft and lower end of the femur are more problematic. Powerful muscles attach to this bone, and spasm of these muscles causes the sharp bone ends to pierce muscle and other soft tissues, causing heavy bleeding. These fractures must be immobilized immediately. If there are extra hands, have one person apply steady traction to the leg by pulling on the foot while another person applies countertraction to the pelvis. Pull until the pain is relieved (this will usually require a force of about 10 percent of the victim's body weight), and maintain traction on the leg while a splint is being applied. One simple technique is to secure the broken leg to the uninjured one. Or you can strap a tree branch, oar, or some other long object to the leg from chest to ankle. But make sure there is padding over all bony prominences, such as the knee and ankle. And put a soft roll under the knee so that it's flexed about 5 or 10 degrees.

If there are six or more people in your party, you can consider transporting the victim out overland. If you don't have the manpower, send someone for a helicopter rescue crew.

Kneecap

This is another one of those unpadded bones. A fractured kneecap can be hard to distinguish from a bad bruise. If there is a lot of swelling over the front of the knee and you feel crepitus when you press down on the kneecap, it's probably broken. The best treatment is a cylindrical splint from groin to ankle. A rolled-up foam sleeping pad will do nicely. Climbing will be almost impossible with this injury, but the victim can walk over gentle terrain with the help of a walking stick.

Lower Leg

A fall from a height may result in a fracture of the upper part of the leg bone (tibia). These fractures usually involve the knee joint, and bleeding will cause the knee to swell like a balloon. Fractures of the shaft of the tibia are frequently angulated and open, and the thin bone that runs alongside the tibia (the fibula) is usually broken also. If the leg is deformed and CMS is impaired, realign the bones by grasping the ankle and applying steady traction along the long axis of the bone until it straightens out. Then splint it. If the bone is protruding, wash the fracture site with antiseptic solution (or soap and water) and apply a sterile dressing or the cleanest cloth bandage available. Then reduce and splint the fracture.

Ankle

Ankle fractures and sprains are often indistinguishable: a swollen, tender ankle could as easily be fractured as sprained. Run your fingers over the bony knob on each side of the ankle, feeling for deformity

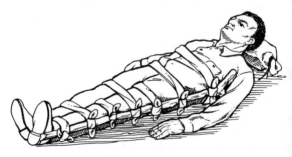

9. *Splinting a fractured leg.*

and crepitus. If you find none, call it a sprain and apply the RICE technique. If ice isn't available, cold water or snow will help to reduce swelling and alleviate pain. The victim may be able to walk with some help. If there is no deformity, it may be better to leave his boot on. It will make an excellent splint, and you'll never get it back on once it has been off for a while.

Fractures of the ankle often come as a package deal with dislocations. These are usually obvious, with the foot discolored and bent at a weird angle. This puts the stretch on the blood vessels in the area, and prompt reduction is necessary to save the foot. Grasp the foot with the heel in one hand and the other hand over the top of the foot, then pull steadily toward you. The ankle will slip back into place with a "thud" and a nice pink color will return to the foot as the circulation returns. A pillow, down parka, or other soft, bulky object wrapped around the ankle and pinned in place makes an excellent splint.

Foot

Jumping from a height and landing on the feet is a recipe for a fractured heel or long bone of the foot (metatarsal). Fractures of the heel are often associated with compression fractures of the spine, so make sure that you examine that area also. Splint suspected fractures of the heel area as you would an ankle fracture. A stiff-soled boot makes a good splint for metatarsal fractures.

Fractured toes heal nicely if you just tape them to their buddies. Put a little cotton between the toes to absorb moisture and prevent skin maceration. There is a great deal of pressure on the big toe during the toe-off phase of walking, so fractures of this digit can be disabling. Stiff-soled boots help to take some pressure off the fracture, especially if you tape four or five tongue depressors across the sole at its widest part.

?❧ DISLOCATIONS

Reducing a dislocated joint can be like trying to put "Jack" back in the box. It's a tough job, but someone has to do it. And quickly. If you don't pop that shoulder (or elbow, finger, or hip) back in right away, swelling and muscle spasm will make the job next to impossible. And reducing the dislocation provides instant pain relief, takes the pressure off the nerves and blood vessels around the joint, and allows you to splint the injured limb in a comfortable position. A wound over a dislocated joint constitutes an "open dislocation." Clean the wound thoroughly and apply a sterile bandage before any attempt to reduce it. *Always* check CMS before and after reduction.

Here are some of the common dislocations encountered in the wilderness and how to handle them:

Dislocated Shoulder

Every outdoorsman should be able to recognize and treat a dislocated shoulder. These are common injuries and relatively easy to reduce. They are usually the result of a backward force on an elevated arm, as illustrated by "Rick," the elk hunter. *Warning:* Before you start yanking on that "dislocated" shoulder, make sure that it really is out of joint. Unless you carry x-ray glasses in your pocket, this can be tricky. But you can be reasonably sure of your diagnosis if

1. The shoulder has an unnatural, "squared-off" appearance.
2. The arm is held out from the body.
3. The victim can't place his hand on the uninjured shoulder.

Here is one way to reduce a dislocated shoulder: Have the victim lie prone on a ledge or other flat surface with the dislocated arm hanging over the edge. Use strips of cloth or other material to secure a weight of 10 to 15 pounds to the wrist. Then take a short hike. When you return in ten minutes, the shoulder will be back in joint.

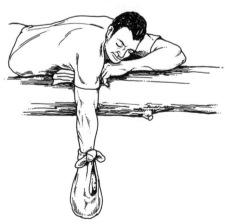

10. *Reducing a dislocated shoulder.*

Here is another technique. Position the victim as above, with the injured arm hanging over an edge. Sit or kneel next to him, wrap your hands around his upper arm, and gently pull down on the upper arm. Gradually increase the downward force on the arm until you feel the shoulder slip back into joint. You'll know when it's back in when you hear the victim give a huge sigh of relief, and a beatific smile spreads across his face.

Immediately after reducing the shoulder, put the arm in a sling and swathe, keeping the hand and wrist free so that you can check the circulation at regular intervals.

Separated Shoulder

One common mistake is to mistake a "separated" shoulder for a dislocation. A separation is generally caused by a fall directly onto the shoulder, causing disruption of the ligaments that connect the collarbone with the shoulder blade (scapula). In a partial separation, the ligaments are only partially torn, and you will find swelling and tenderness over the end of the collarbone. In a complete separation, the ligaments are totally disrupted, and the end of the collarbone is elevated an inch or more. (You can distinguish between a separation and a fractured collarbone by pressing over the end of the collarbone. If it feels "springy," you are dealing with a separation. If the collarbone is very tender and feels "crunchy," it's fractured.) Separated shoulders should be immobilized in a sling. (Complete separations sometimes require surgery to restore normal function of the shoulder in an active, athletic person.)

Elbow

You will know a dislocated elbow when you see one. A hard fall on the arm drives the forearm bones backward and out of the elbow joint. These dislocations can be tough to reduce, but worth a try if you are more than a few hours from help. Pull slowly and steadily on the forearm while an assistant pulls in the opposite direction on the upper arm. You will feel the elbow go back in, and the victim will be able to bend it to 90 degrees. If one or two good efforts fail to reduce the dislocation, put the arm in a sling and hit the trail. Undue force will only result in unnecessary pain and in damage to the joint and nerves and blood vessels.

Finger

Dislocations of the first joint of the finger are common on wilderness treks, usually the result of the finger being struck and bent back by a thrown object. A dislocated finger is always obvious. Reduce it by pulling straight out on the deformed digit with one hand while pushing the base of the dislocated bone back into joint with the thumb of your other hand. Then splint the finger to its buddy.

Hip

It takes a fall off a cliff or a similar violent injury to dislocate the hip, a very stable "ball-and-socket" joint. Either the thigh will be sticking out at an odd angle, or the leg will be shortened, rotated inward, and crossed over the uninjured leg.

While reducing a dislocated hip in the wild is no mean feat, it should be attempted. The longer the hip is out of the socket, the greater the risk of complications, including damage to the sciatic nerve and necrosis of the ball part of the joint. Lay the victim supine on the ground and slowly bend the knee and hip to 90 degrees so that the knee and foot are pointing up. Have an assistant push down on the hips while you straddle the victim, place his leg between your thighs, and wrap your hands behind his knee. Then pull up hard on his thigh while you gently rotate the leg first one way and then the other. When you feel the hip go in, splint it to the other leg with soft padding between the knees. If you cannot reduce it, splint it in a comfortable position and arrange to evacuate the victim.

Kneecaps

Scrambling down a rocky mountainside can cause a sudden twisting motion of the knee that can dislocate the kneecap. A direct blow to the inner side of the kneecap will do the trick, too. The kneecap will be displaced laterally, and the knee will be flexed 45 or 60 degrees. These dislocations can usually be reduced by slowly straightening the knee. You may have to gently nudge the kneecap back into place by pressing laterally on it with your hand. When it's reduced, apply a cylindrical splint to keep the knee in a fully straightened position. Walking may be a little painful, but it is safe.

~~ **AMPUTATIONS**

Amputations are treated the same way as an open fracture. Control bleeding by holding firm pressure over the stump with a bandage or rolled-up clothing. Then irrigate it with disinfected water before applying a sterile dressing secured with an elastic bandage. The amputated part should be cleaned and transported with the victim. Cover it with a moistened, sterile bandage, and put it in a plastic bag, filled with ice if possible.

HEADS UP:
HEAD AND NECK
INJURIES IN THE WILD

It had been a long hike up the old logging road to the pristine lake high in Idaho's Salmon National Forest. But it had been worth it. Between them, Jim and Ron had landed a half dozen goldens in the first hour after sunrise. But now it was time to return to camp on the Lehmi River, 2,000 feet below. They dreaded the long hike down. The trail was a tedious series of switchbacks, like a long row of ribbon candy stretching down the mountain. They decided to take a dangerous but much quicker trail down the boulder-studded back side of the mountain.

They started picking their way down the precipitous rock face. Jim slid on the seat of his pants down the side of one large boulder, and sat on a ledge and waited for his partner. He didn't have to wait long. Ron lost his footing and let out a blood-curdling yell as he went tumbling head over heels down the mountainside. He came to a stop sixty bruising yards later at the bottom of a steep defile. Jim leaned over the ledge and peered down into the gorge. All he could see were Ron's legs. They weren't moving. His eyes moved farther down the slope. Far below he could just make out a narrow ribbon of white water: the Lehmi River. It was a long way off.

ॐ

Jim is caught on a rock in a high place. His buddy just took a bad tumble, and is either unconscious, paralyzed from a spinal injury, or both. And he may have fractures and internal injuries as well. Jim has to get Ron out of there, but if he tries to move him without immobilizing his neck, he could do irreparable harm to his spinal cord. So what should he do? Would you know what to do? Let's go through the systematic series of steps that you would need to take to get your partner and yourself off that mountain.

?◆ BACK TO BASICS

The approach to the badly injured person has got to be streamlined and efficient. Start with the "ABCs": *a*irway, *b*reathing, and *c*irculation, as described in Chapter 1. Once you have attended to any immediately life-threatening problems, assess his mental status by evaluating the following areas:

1. *Eye opening:* Does he open his eyes spontaneously, or only on command or in response to a painful stimulus?
2. *Verbal response:* Is his speech understandable, and does he make sense? Or is he confused and disoriented, or talking gibberish?
3. *Motor response:* Does he obey simple commands? Does he withdraw from a painful stimulus?

Then check the pupils. They should be symmetrical and react to light by constricting. Confusion, lethargy, garbled speech, and unequal or unreactive pupils are all signs of possible brain injury.

The next step is to resuscitate the trauma victim with the materials at hand. He might need oxygen, intravenous fluids, blood transfusion, antibiotics, and a urinary catheter, but if it's just you and him on a rocky crag, you're not going to be able to do much more than to make him comfortable and perhaps give him a drink of water. (And if he has a serious head injury, fluids by mouth are out because he could aspirate them into his lungs.)

?◆ CHECK THE SPINE

As you do your head-to-toe exam, check for signs of spinal fractures. Remember: any blow to the head, face, or neck and any fall from a significant height can produce a spinal injury. The golden rule of spinal injuries is: every trauma victim has one until proved otherwise. And if he does have a fracture or fracture-dislocation of the spine, the slightest movement can drive sharp fragments of bone into the spinal cord, resulting in permanent paralysis or death.

Ask the victim if he has pain in his neck or back. Then, without moving him, slip your hand between the ground and his back and run your fingers down his spinal column from the base of the skull to the base of spine, feeling for tenderness or any abnormal prominence. If there is any sign of a neck injury, immobilize the neck by placing "sandbags" (sacks stuffed with dirt or tightly bundled clothing) around his neck, head, and shoulders. The "sandbags" can

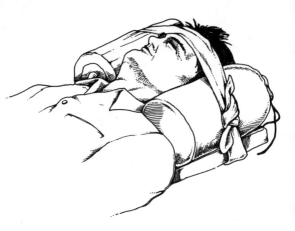

11. Immobilizing the neck.

then be anchored in place with rocks, or a strip of adhesive tape can be drawn across his forehead and secured to the bags on either side. If you suspect a back injury, keep the victim in a supine position.

After immobilizing the spine, look for a *spinal cord injury*. These are the signs:

1. Pain in the neck or back radiating down the arms or legs.
2. Numbness or tingling in the hands or feet.
3. Loss of sensation in the arms or legs.
4. Paralysis of the arms or legs.
5. A sustained penile erection ("priapism").

?➍ HEADS UP

With head injuries, what you see is not always what you get. It's hard not to get excited when your buddy hits his head on a rock overhang and lays his scalp open down to the bone. The bleeding can be horrendous, and he may turn pale and feel punk for a while. But that doesn't mean that he has a brain injury. On the other hand, he could have serious bleeding *inside* the skull with nary a mark on his scalp. Of far greater importance than the appearance of the scalp is his mental state. Was he knocked unconscious? Is he awake and alert now? Is he oriented to his surroundings, or does he think he's on the planet Tralfalmador? Check his orientation to person, place, and time. Then decide whether he has one of the following injuries:

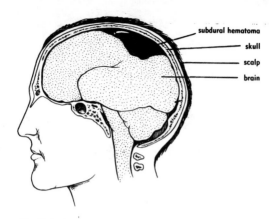

12. Subudural hematoma.

Concussion

You don't have to be a neurosurgeon to treat most brain injuries in the wild. That's because most of these injuries are simple *concussions*. A concussion is a transient disturbance of brain function following a blow to the head. The hallmark of a concussion is a brief loss of consciousness, often followed by a period of mild confusion, memory loss, headache, and perhaps some nausea and vomiting. These symptoms resolve within a few hours or days at the most.

Intracranial Bleeding

You *do* have to be a neurosurgeon to treat a blood clot on the brain (*subdural* or *epidural hematoma*). Any blow to the head, especially over the relatively thin part of the skull just above the ear, can cause a tear in the vessels in or under the covering of the brain (the dura). Because the skull is a rigid compartment, there's no room for expansion. So when a vessel on the surface of the brain bleeds, it forms a clot that increases the pressure within the skull. When the pressure becomes great enough, blood flow to the brain ceases and the brain dies. It's "thanks for the memories," unless something is done to relieve the pressure. That means immediate evacuation to a hospital.

The person who develops a blood clot on the brain may be knocked unconscious and never regain consciousness. Or he may regain consciousness for a brief period (the "lucid interval"), only to lapse back into unconsciousness. And occasionally (especially in older people) there is no initial loss of consciousness, but increasing confusion and lethargy progressing to coma some hours or days after the injury.

How do you know when your buddy has a life-threatening clot on the brain? Unless there's a CT scanner there in the woods, you won't know. You're going to have to keep a close eye on him for at least 24 hours, observing for

- Personality changes.
- Vomiting.
- Increasing headache.
- Unequal pupils. If one pupil becomes widely dilated, he has a very serious problem. The brain is being squeezed out of the skull, and the situation is desperate.

Other things to look for include

- Dropping pulse rate. As the pressure in the head rises, the blood pressure goes up and the heart rate slows.
- Blood or clear fluid draining from the ears or nose. This may be a sign of a fracture of the base of the skull.
- Obvious fracture or indentation of the skull. Run your fingers through the hair, feeling for fractures, depressed areas, and lacerations.
- Bruises behind the ears and "raccoon eyes" (also signs of a fractured skull).
- Spinal injury. Fifteen percent of victims of severe head injury also have a broken neck. If the victim is unconscious, assume he has a broken neck and immobilize his head.

Scalp wounds can bleed like Old Faithful. The best way to control the bleeding is to sew them up. If you don't have the wherewithal, here's an alternative that doesn't require needle and thread: Clean the wound, irrigating it with the cleanest water available, and pick out dirt particles, sticks, and so on. Then moisten the hair on either side of the laceration and twist small clumps of hair into knots all along the wound edges. Tie these braids across the wound until it's closed up tight. Then apply a turban dressing with a few rolls of gauze or cloth. The wound will have to be explored and closed under sterile conditions later, but this technique will control bleeding in the meantime. (*Warning:* If there is an obvious skull fracture, *don't* irrigate the wound. That would only drive dirt and bacteria into the brain. Just apply a sterile dressing and a bulky bandage. If there is an arrow, rock, or other foreign object embedded in the skull, *don't touch it!* Doing so could result in cata-strophic bleeding into the brain. Apply a bandage to the wound with the object in place.)

✤ EVACUATION

When do you evacuate the head injury victim? You can best make this judgment by assigning him to one of three risk groups:

1. *Low risk:* The victim has sustained a mild blow to the head, but had no loss of consciousness, and complains only of a minor headache and dizzi-ness. He may have a small laceration or bruise on the scalp, but his pupils are symmetrical and he has no paralysis, loss of sensation, or other sign of neurologic injury.
2. *Moderate risk:* The victim has had a brief loss of consciousness, vomiting, persistent or worsening headache, and amnesia for the events immediately following the injury.
3. *High risk:* The victim was knocked unconscious and now has a depressed level of consciousness or loss of sensation or strength on one side of the body. Anyone who has fallen more than fifteen feet, who has sustained a high-energy blow from a falling rock or other object, or who has suffered a skull fracture or penetrating injury to the skull should be considered at high risk, even if there was no loss of consciousness or other sign of brain injury.

Those who fall into the "low-risk" group can be expected to do well, but should be watched carefully for 24 hours. They will need to be evacuated if they develop signs of lethargy, drowsiness, personality change, forceful or persistent vomiting, or abnormal gait or speech. Those in the "high-risk" category need to be evaluated in a hospital, and must be evac-uated as quickly as possible. The disposition of those in the "moderate-risk" group depends on a number of factors, including other injuries and evacuation time. Generally, anyone in this category who also has spinal or other injuries should be evacuated at once.

How about the person with a neck or spinal in-jury? If he has only minimal pain in the neck or back, and there's no sign of paralysis, he can safely walk out under his own power. If he has significant pain but no sign of a spinal cord injury, keep him immobilized and recheck him every 20 minutes. Subtle signs of spinal cord injury may become apparent only after repeated exams. If there are *definite* signs of a spinal cord injury, go for help. Any attempt to move the victim at this point can result in catastrophe.

Evacuating an unconscious person out of the mountains or deep woods can be one of the Labors of Hercules, so hit the trail while the victim is still awake and able to cooperate in his evacuation. If he is reasonably alert, he can walk without assistance. But keep a close eye on him, especially when going over rough terrain that may require normal balance and judgment.

If you have enough strong people in your party, it may be best to evacuate an unconscious person yourselves. But make sure that his neck is rigidly immobilized if there is any possibility of spinal injury. Carry him supine on a litter with the head slightly elevated to help increase the drainage of venous blood from the brain and to reduce swelling. If he vomits, lower his head and turn him on his side so that he doesn't aspirate the vomited material into his lungs. (If his spine is immobilized, logroll him over onto his side.) And make sure that you put padding under his shoulders, elbows, buttocks, and heels to prevent pressure sores.

Rescuing a head- or neck-injured victim in the wild may be the toughest challenge you will ever face. It calls for all the stamina, courage, and ingenuity you possess, but your buddy will thank you.

CHEST AND ABDOMINAL INJURIES

Charlie couldn't believe his luck. Here it was only the first day, heck, the first hour of bow season, and already a hefty buck, a nine-pointer at least, had emerged from the panoply of mustard- and cinnamon-colored leaves at the edge of the clearing and stood sniffing the wet morning air. He was an easy target. All Charlie had to do was quietly draw the bow up to his cheek, pull back steadily on the arrow, and let it fly to its target. And he did. The arrow struck home just behind the buck's shoulder, and the shocked animal turned and staggered into the deep cover.

Charlie let out a whoop and started to climb down from the tree stand, holding the compound bow in his left hand. He was reaching for a branch when the one he was standing on suddenly snapped, and he fell to the ground. He landed on his left side, right on the business end of an arrow. It penetrated his chest just below his left nipple. Charlie let out an anguished scream, then rolled over onto his back. He lay there for a moment, fighting panic and a wall of pain, convinced he was going to die.

 ॰

Charlie is in trouble. Any serious chest or abdominal wound spells trouble in the wilderness. And they happen. Even if Charlie had not landed on an arrow, he probably would have sustained a blunt chest or abdominal injury after falling from that tree. He could easily have broken a few ribs, which in turn could have caused a collapsed lung, bleeding into his chest cavity, flail chest, and any number of other complications, including a lacerated liver or spleen. It's not hard to slip while crossing mountainous or rocky terrain, and it seems as though there is always a tree stump, tent pole, ice axe, or some other pointed object waiting to skewer you in the chest as you tumble to the ground.

Many of these blunt or penetrating chest and abdominal injuries are life-threatening, and require immediate evacuation. But some can be treated adequately in the field. Let's talk about how you size up such injuries in the wild and what you can do to treat them or stabilize them while preparing for evacuation.

?? CHEST INJURIES

The chest is a bellows, which Webster defines as "a machine that by alternate expansion and contraction draws in air through a valve or orifice and expels it through a tube." When the chest muscles and diaphragm (the broad, flat muscle that separates the chest and abdominal cavities) contract, the chest expands, creating negative pressure in the chest cavity. Air rushes into the lungs through the mouth and respiratory tree for a few seconds, and then is expelled as the chest muscles relax. Chest injuries have to be understood in terms of their effect on the chest bellows. Any injury that violates the integrity of the chest wall or causes an obstruction of the respiratory tree will make breathing difficult or impossible, and then it's "curtains for certain," unless you intervene to set things right in a hurry.

?? EVALUATING CHEST WOUNDS

Unless you have fluoroscopic glasses, you're going to have to rely on your senses of sight, touch, and hearing to evaluate a chest injury in the wild. But the signs of serious chest injury are rarely subtle. Physical diagnosis is based on the examiner's ability to inspect, feel, percuss, and listen for signs of disease or injury. Here's a crash course in the examination of the chest:

Inspect

As with any trauma victim, first check to make sure that he has an adequate airway and that he is breathing. Count the number of breaths per minute, and note the breathing pattern. The normal breathing rate at rest is 12 to 20 breaths a minute. Very slow, fast, or irregular breathing denotes trouble. How is his color? If he's blue, he's not breathing effectively. Look at the neck. Are the veins distended? That may be a sign of a "tension pneumothorax" (see below). Is the trachea (windpipe) in the center of the neck or pushed over to one side (another sign of tension pneumothorax)? Expose the chest and look for abrasions, lacerations, puncture wounds, or asymmetrical movement.

Feel

Gently run your hands over the chest, from the collarbones down to the abdomen, and from the breastbone to the backbone. Take note of any tender areas, signifying broken or contused ribs or breastbone. If there is a crunchy feeling over the bone, it's probably fractured. A bubbly feeling under the skin (subcutaneous crepitus) is a sure sign of a collapsed lung. What you're feeling is air that has leaked out of the lung and percolated into the tissues under the skin. You might feel crepitus anywhere from the neck to the groin.

Percuss

Place your long finger at various points on the chest wall and tap the end of it with the long finger of your other hand. You should hear a slightly hollow sound from the collarbones to about the sixth rib in the front, and from the shoulder blades to about the tenth rib in the back. Don't worry about the exact pitch of the sound that you hear as you percuss. The important thing to look for is marked differences from one side to the other. A *very* hollow percussion note indicates collapse of the lung, while a very dull sound indicates a chest cavity filled with blood (hemothorax).

Listen

Put your ear to first one side of the chest and then the other, and have the victim take several deep breaths. You should hear the sound of air moving into and out of each lung. A loud, harsh sound on one or both sides indicates obstruction of the upper airway. A wheezing or rattling sound suggests blood or fluid in the bronchial tubes or air sacs. The absence of sound on one side means that air is not moving into that lung, because of either a collapsed lung or a chest cavity filled with blood.

?➥ BLUNT CHEST INJURY

Rib Fractures

A fall onto a rock, log, or other hard surface can crack a rib or two. These are painful injuries, and hurt more with deep inspiration. Run your fingers over the injured area. A tender area with underlying crepitus most likely represents a fractured rib. You can confirm the diagnosis by pressing down on the breastbone with the victim in the supine position. If he complains of pain in a rib, it's fractured.

An uncomplicated rib fracture is a painful but not disabling injury if the pain can be controlled. But be wary of fractures of the first three ribs and the lower ribs on either side. They are often associated with injuries to the great vessels and to the liver and spleen, respectively. And multiple fractured ribs should alert you to the possibility of serious underlying injury to the lung, heart, vessels, or abdominal organs. These people need to be evacuated.

Treatment of a simple rib fracture requires nothing more than a bottle of aspirin or some other analgesic. Rib belts and taping of the ribs may give marginal pain relief, but they restrict movement of the rib cage, causing underventilation of the lung. This can lead to pneumonia and other complications.

Separated Cartilage

The ribs don't join directly to the breastbone. Instead, they connect to a short segment of cartilage which then joins the breastbone. A hard blow to the front of the chest can cause a disruption of this rib-cartilage junction, or "separated cartilage." These are very painful injuries which are hard to distinguish from fractured ribs. Treatment is the same.

Fractured Breastbone

It's not easy to break the breastbone. It requires the kind of high-energy impact you'd get from falling off a cliff or ramming a snowmobile into a tree at high speed. There will be tenderness and crepitus over the breastbone, and the chest may have a caved-in appearance. These are serious injuries and are often associated with contusions of the heart and lacerations of the lung. Attend to the ABC's and arrange for rapid medical evacuation. The victim will be able to breathe more easily in an upright position (this is true of any chest injury).

Flail Chest

When three or more consecutive ribs are each fractured in two or more places, there will be an unstable segment of chest wall. This is known as a "flail chest." You can diagnose this injury by looking for "paradoxical" movement of the chest wall in the area of the injury: when the rest of the chest is expanding, the negative pressure in the chest cavity will pull in on the "floating" flail segment, and positive pressure will cause it to move outward with expiration. Obviously, this interferes with normal breathing. And the lung tissue under the flail segment is often contused or lacerated. Classically, these injuries are tolerated fairly well for a day or two, and then the victim goes into respiratory failure, often requiring artificial ventilation for a while. Old medical textbooks recommend splinting and bolstering the flail segment with tape, hooks, and sandbags; but these just make things worse. Give him analgesics and get him out of there before he deteriorates.

Pneumothorax

When air enters the chest cavity through a hole in the chest wall, or a fractured rib pokes a hole in the lung, pressure rises in the chest cavity until the lung collapses. This is a pneumothorax. The victim will be short of breath, breath sounds will be diminished on the affected side, and you'll hear a hollow sound when you percuss over the collapsed lung. These are painful injuries, but he may be able to walk out of the woods under his own power. All but small pneumothoraces require insertion of a chest tube to drain air from the chest cavity. You won't be doing this in the wilderness unless your name is De Bakey and you brought along a chest tube.

Tension Pneumothorax

When air leaks from a punctured lung into the chest cavity but can't escape, that side of the chest will fill up with air. The pressure increases to the point that the heart, great vessels, windpipe, and other midline structures are pushed over to the opposite side of the chest. The great veins in the chest become kinked, and venous blood can't return to the heart. The victim turns blue, the neck veins become engorged, and cardiovascular collapse ensues. This is called a tension pneumothorax. Death is imminent if the chest isn't decompressed immediately. (*Warning:* This technique requires a large, sterile needle and proper training.) The needle is inserted into the space between the second and third ribs at any point lateral to the nipple. Guide the needle over the top of the third rib and then perpendicularly down into the chest until you hear a gush of air as the needle enters the chest cavity. The victim's appearance will improve dramatically after this procedure, but he's still not out of danger. Leave the needle in place, and make arrangements for a hasty evacuation to a hospital where a chest tube can be inserted.

Hemothorax

Rib fractures can cause bleeding from the artery that runs along the undersurface of the rib or from a punctured lung. The blood collects in the chest cavity, causing a hemothorax. The victim will be hurtin' for certain, and short of breath. If you tap over the affected side, it will sound dull. An isolated hemothorax is not an immediate life-threatening injury. Blood loss into the chest cavity is rarely enough to cause shock, and respiratory distress is usually not severe. There's nothing you can do for the guy with hemothorax except to make him as comfortable as possible while awaiting evacuation.

?❧ PENETRATING CHEST WOUNDS

An arrow in the chest can ruin your deer season. Every year there are reports of hunters impaling themselves on arrows when they slip climbing out of tree stands. (The correct technique is to tie a line to the bow and lower it to the ground before climbing down.) Other outdoorsmen transfix themselves on ski poles, ice axes, or tent poles. This is serious business. Even if the offending object misses the heart, lungs, and great vessels (an unlikely proposition), at the very least it's going to poke a hole in the chest wall and create a pneumothorax or hemopneumothorax. And if it punctures the chest below the nipple line, there's an excellent chance that it will skewer the liver, spleen, or other abdominal organs.

In the old Indian movies, they'd just yank the arrow out of the guy's chest and he'd be all set to return to the action. That's *not* the thing to do. The impaling object has created a channel through the tissues. But as long as it occupies that channel, bleeding will be controlled by the "tamponading" effect it has on torn blood vessels. Always leave the arrow, pole, or what have you exactly where it is.

One of the most dangerous chest wounds is the *sucking chest wound*. If the hole in the chest wall approaches the diameter of the windpipe, it becomes impossible for the bellows mechanism to create negative pressure in the chest cavity, and the lungs won't expand. Instead, air is sucked through the hole in the chest into the chest cavity. It's like trying to run a vacuum cleaner with a large hole in the canister.

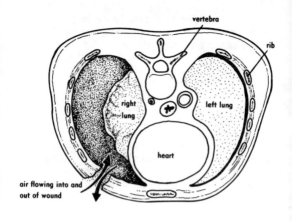

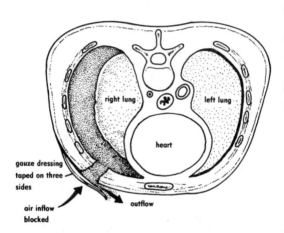

13. Sucking chest wound.

You have to act fast when confronted with a sucking chest wound. Cover it with the cleanest bandage available—a shirt, a towel, or even your hand if necessary. After the victim is stabilized you can take the time to apply a sterile, petrolatum gauze (Adaptic, for example) dressing right over the wound, and cover it with a sterile 4 × 4 gauze pad. Tape the pad on three sides, so that air can escape but not enter through the wound. (If you seal it up tight, you'll create a tension pneumothorax. That's considered bad form.) As with any chest wound, these people have to be medically evacuated out ASAP.

⁊❧ ABDOMINAL INJURIES

Blunt Abdominal Injuries

Blunt abdominal injuries are rarely as dramatic or immediately life-threatening as chest injuries. But they can be just as deadly. It's rare for a chest injury to lead to hemorrhagic shock. But you can easily lose a couple of quarts of blood from a ruptured spleen or liver. As blood collects in the rigid chest cavity, the pressure within the cavity increases until the bleeding vessels are "tamponaded." But as blood collects in the abdominal cavity, the abdominal wall stretches, and impressive amounts of blood can be lost before pressure rises within the cavity. By then, it may be too late to do anything about it if you're in the wilderness.

The tricky thing about blunt abdominal injuries is that they are rarely obvious. These injuries are hard enough to diagnose in a hospital setting with high-tech diagnostic equipment, let alone in the deep woods when all you have to work with is your brain, your eyes, and your hands. The key is to know when to look for these injuries, and then to examine the victim carefully at repeat intervals. Obviously, if your buddy slips and falls belly-down on a tree stump, you're going to think about blunt abdominal trauma. But you should also think about blunt abdominal trauma if he cracks his breastbone or a few lower ribs. Pain in both the abdomen and the left shoulder should also alert you to a ruptured spleen.

First, look for signs of shock: thready pulse, blue fingertips, cold, clammy skin, agitation, and rapid breathing. Then gently roll him onto his back, and expose his abdomen. Note any bruises or discoloration, and check for rib fractures. Is his belly soft, or are his muscles rigid? Gently press under the rib cage on the right (liver) and left (spleen), the pit of the stomach, and both lower quadrants. A bruised abdominal wall may cause localized tenderness, but if you find persistent rigidity and tenderness, along with signs of early shock, you've got to assume that he has a blunt injury. Treat him like any shock victim and prepare to evacuate him. (A swollen, tight abdominal wall is a very late sign of abdominal bleeding and will be accompanied by signs of late shock.)

A blow to the flank or the back can injure the kidneys. The hallmark of a contused or ruptured kidney is blood in the urine (hematuria). If the kidney is just contused, the hematuria will stop within a few hours. If the kidney is lacerated or ruptured, it may continue to bleed, causing persistent hematuria and, eventually, signs of shock. Treat the shock and prepare to evacuate the victim.

Penetrating Abdominal Injuries

You don't have to be a surgeon to diagnose a penetrating abdominal injury. There are usually plenty of clues. These are the important things to keep in mind:

1. Any wound from the nipple line to the groin can involve the abdominal contents.
2. Gunshot exit wounds are larger than entrance wounds. Look for exit wounds by examining the back, chest, and legs.
3. A shotgun blast at close range can create a big defect in the abdominal wall, causing bowel to protrude through the wound. *Don't replace it!* Stool will soil the abdominal cavity, causing peritonitis. Just cover eviscerated bowel with moist dressings.
4. These injuries need prompt surgical exploration and repair. Apply sterile dressings to all wounds and evacuate the victim as quickly as possible.

7

EYE, EAR, NOSE, AND THROAT PROBLEMS

❧ THE EYES HAVE IT: EYE INJURIES IN THE WILD

Poets call the eye the "window to the soul." True enough. But the eye is much more than that. It's also a sophisticated camera, with a dust cover (eyelids), a lens system, a variable aperture system (pupil and iris), and "film" (retina). We're not talking Instamatic here. The human eye is "high tech," with features you won't find in those fancy Japanese cameras—like automatic focus, depth perception, an automatic light meter, and voluntary and involuntary fixation systems and "pursuit movement" that allows us to (1) look for grouse in a barberry thicket, (2) keep an eye on him while he's trying to decide whether to sit tight or run for it, and (3) lock onto the grouse when it flushes.

You've got to take care of optical equipment like that when you're running around out in the woods. And there's a lot more to it than dodging swinging branches. Your eyes are vulnerable to a wide range of injuries in the outdoors, everything from frozen corneas to solar retinitis. Let's take a look at a few of these ocular hazards.

Corneal Foreign Bodies and Abrasions

These are the most common eye injuries in the wild. The cornea is the clear membrane that overlies the iris, the colored part of the eye. The nerve endings are packed in there like fly fishermen on a prime trout stream on opening day, making it the most sensitive structure in the human body. When the wind blows a grain of sand in your eye it can feel like a needle. It will make your eyes water and your lids snap shut like the jaws of a bear trap. Most often, tears will wash out sand and other foreign bodies. That's the good news. The bad news is that they are

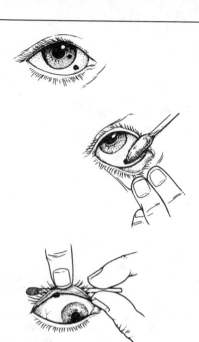

14. Removing a foreign body from the eye.

sometimes caught under the upper lid, and are dragged back and forth across the cornea a few times before they are washed away, leaving you with a painful corneal abrasion. The important thing to know about a corneal abrasion is that it feels *exactly* like a corneal foreign body.

Here is what you do if sand, grit, or embers blow into your eye: Have your buddy take a good look at the eye. He should first check the shape and symmetry of the pupils and do a rough vision check (he should ask you to count fingers or read newsprint). Then he should search carefully for foreign bodies, checking the cornea, under both lids, and in the corners. (Use a Q-tip or a match stem to evert the upper lid, a favorite hiding place for grit.) If he sees something, he should try to flush it out with a gentle stream of clean water. If that doesn't do it, pull the upper lid down over the lashes of the lower lid. Or he can use a Q-tip or the corner of a piece of cloth to lift a piece of sand off the cornea or conjunctiva (see Figure 14).

If the pain persists, you probably have a corneal abrasion. Cover the eye with a tight eye patch for 12 to 24 hours and avoid bright light. If the eye is still painful after being patched for 24 hours, there may be a small particle embedded in the cornea. It will have to be removed by a physician as soon as possible.

Blunt Injury to the Eye

The eye is set back in a protective bony casement, but swinging branches, flying rocks, and fists all can inflict devastating damage. Lacerations, puncture wounds, and contusions are usually obvious. A *hyphema* is bleeding in the front chamber of the eye, just behind the cornea. It can lead to glaucoma and blood staining of the cornea. Fluid in the back chamber of the eye seeping through a tear in the retina causes the thin retina to peel off the back of the eye like loose wall paper. This is known as a *detached retina*. A *dislocated lens* is usually pushed backward, but you may see it in the front chamber of the eye.

These are all severe, vision-threatening injuries. There is not much you can do about them except to gently wash dirt and debris away from the eye with disinfected warm water, cover *both* eyes with opaque eye shields (to minimize eye movement), and evacuate the victim to the nearest medical facility. *Never* attempt to remove a foreign body that is embedded inside the eyeball. If a fishhook, thorn, or some other large object is embedded in the eye, do *not* attempt to remove it. Prevent further damage by taping a styrofoam or paper cup over the eye, then evacuate to the nearest hospital.

Snow Blindness

Snow blindness is sunburn of the corneas. You're more likely to get it at high altitudes, where ultraviolet radiation (UVR) is more intense (4 percent increase in intensity for each 300 meters increase in altitude) and where snow and ice reflect up to 85 percent of incident UVR into your eyes. UVR in the UVB range (290–320 manometers) is absorbed by the thin layer of cells on the surface of the cornea. (UVA is transmitted to the lens, where it can cause cataracts over a period of time.) These cells swell and rupture, and the cornea becomes hazy. You won't realize what's going on for 6 to 12 hours. Then your eyes will begin to water and redden, your lids will swell, and you'll feel as though you have hot cinders in your eyes.

Snow blindness is temporary, and the corneas heal spontaneously in about 24 hours. But there are some things you can do to relieve the pain. First, remove contact lenses. Then, apply cold compresses to the eyes. When things have simmered down a little, apply tight patches to both eyes for 12 to 24 hours. But you don't really want to be knocking around in the mountains with your eyes patched. Some of those crevices are pretty deep. So avoid the problem altogether by wearing sunglasses (more on eyewear later). If you forget your sunglasses, you can fashion a crude pair by cutting narrow slits in cardboard or some other material and strapping it to your head with string or elastic.

Frozen Cornea

This is a wind-chill injury. You can get it by trying to force your eyes open while walking into a stiff breeze on a very cold day or while riding a snowmobile. The symptoms are similar to those of a corneal injury or snow blindness: blurred vision, red, watery eyes, lid spasm, and sensitivity to light. There is no pain, however, until the corneas start to rewarm. Treatment consists of rapid rewarming with warm (104 degrees) compresses and patching for several hours.

Solar Retinitis

Solar retinitis is what you get when you stare at the sun, especially during a solar eclipse. The lens of the eye acts as a magnifying glass, focusing an intense beam of light on the retina. It can actually burn a hole in the retina, causing a permanent blind spot in the center of your visual field.

Contact Lenses

Contact lens wearers know about the contact lens corollary to Murphy's law: Anything that *can* go wrong with contact lenses *will* go wrong at the worst possible time. Like the lens that pops out when you're trying to land a trophy lake trout, or the lens that becomes "lost" somewhere in your eyeball just as that 12-point buck starts ambling by your tree stand. But you shouldn't have any problems if you remember the basics of contact lens care and handling. Always wash your hands before handling the lenses, store them in the prescribed manner, don't wear them for longer periods than you would at home, and don't put a scratched or damaged lens in your eye.

The first place to look for a "lost" lens is in the

eye. It may drift off the cornea and under one of the lids. If you don't see it, it's not in the eye. (Contrary to common belief, contact lenses can't slide into the back of the eyeball and pass into the brain. The conjunctiva, the clear membrane that covers the white part of the eye, folds back on itself at the periphery of the eyeball, forming a *cul-de-sac*, or blind pouch, which prevents that from happening.)

The cornea gets oxygen directly from the air, so if you are hunting elk in the high Rockies, or fishing for goldens in some high lake in the Sierra Nevadas where the air is thinner, you may have to cut back on your wearing time.

It is important to remove contact lenses from the eyes of anyone who is unconscious. Remove a soft lens by gently pinching the lens between two fingers and lifting it off. Remove a hard lens by placing a finger on the outer corner of the eye and pulling outward. The lens will pop out.

Sunglasses

Before you go out and buy those new hiking boots or spinning rod, invest a few bucks in the health of your eyes. Get yourself a good pair of sunglasses to protect yourself from snow blindness, cataracts, wind, dust, and glare. You'll need a pair that blocks out 90 percent of visible light, and close to 100 percent of UVR. Glass, polycarbonate, and plastic each have advantages and disadvantages which you can discuss with your optician. You can also ask him about "gradient" and photochromic lenses. Polarizing lenses reduce the glare from snowfields and lake surfaces. Lens color is a matter of personal preference. The frames should be metal, silicone-graphite, nylon, or some other durable material, not plastic.

And don't forget your regular glasses. Plastic lenses absorb 90 percent of UVR, glass lenses about 80 percent. That's good, but you can now buy lenses that block out virtually all UVR. Or you can have your optician treat your current lenses with a UVR filtering dye.

ꝋ EAR, NOSE, AND THROAT DISORDERS

Swimmer's Ear

This is a bacterial infection of the outer ear canal. It is common during the summer months because heat and constant moisture break down the natural barriers to infection in the inner part of the external ear canal. Swimming, frequent showers, and mechanical trauma all predispose to infection with strep and pseudomonas bacteria. Swimmer's ear can cause a sense of fullness in the ear, diminished hearing, intense earache, and a soupy yellow-white discharge. Pulling on the earlobe causes intense pain.

Treatment of swimmer's ear starts with careful irrigation of the canal, injecting sterile water through a bulb syringe or plastic syringe. Then instill several drops of vinegar or Burow's solution four times a day with a medicine dropper. Antibiotic drops are even better, if you happen to have a bottle. You can avoid swimmer's ear by keeping the ears dry, not using earplugs or Q-tips, and by instilling a little vinegar and rubbing alcohol in the ears after each swim or shower.

Dizziness

"Dizziness" means different things to different people. But if you feel as though you are on a merry-go-round (vertigo) every time you lift or turn your head, there is a good chance that you have *labyrinthitis*. This is a short-lived disorder of the organs of balance in the inner ear. It usually lags a head cold by a few days, and may be accompanied by nausea and vomiting. Meclizine, 25 mg three or four times a day, is the treatment of choice.

Ruptured Eardrum

It's not hard to get poked in the ear with a branch while working your way through a grouse covert. If the branch perforates the eardrum, you will have sudden, intense pain in the ear, vertigo, hearing loss, and bleeding from the ear. The branch may have damaged the small bones (ossicles) in the middle ear, so the ear should be examined by a physician as soon as practicable.

If you get cuffed on the ear during a tussle with your buddy, and notice a loss of hearing and bleeding from the ear, the eardrum is probably perforated. In these situations, the eardrum usually heals nicely if left alone. Never put *anything* in the ear if a perforated eardrum is suspected.

A blow to the ear can cause a pool of blood (hematoma) to collect under the skin of the auricle. A large hematoma will lead to "cauliflower ears" if it is not drained. Cleanse the skin with antiseptic solution, then insert a sterile needle into the center of the hematoma and drain as much of the blood as possible. Then apply a compression bandage and an ice bag to the ear.

Few things are as maddening as the feel and sound of an insect crawling around inside your ear. Resist the temptation to squash the bug with a Q-tip. That just creates a mess and can lead to a ruptured eardrum. Instead, take the kinder, gentler approach, and have your buddy flush the critter out with a syringe and some warm water.

Nosebleed

Most nosebleeds will stop if you sit up, lean forward, and squeeze the soft part of the nose for 10 or 15 minutes. Don't lie back or extend your neck. Blood will flow down the back of your throat, nauseating you and making it hard for you to breathe. Persistent bleeding may be related to high blood pressure or may be coming from the back of the nose. Blood loss from a nosebleed can lead to shock. Evacuate to a hospital if you can't stop the bleeding in a reasonable period of time.

Food Caught in the Throat

We talked about "cafe coronaries" in Chapter 1. A piece of meat can go down the right way and *still* give you fits. Large pieces of meat or bread can get hung up in the esophagus and can cause terrific spasms. More than one patient has been admitted to the hospital with the diagnosis of heart attack, when all he really had was a hunk of filet mignon stuck in his esophagus.

If you have a piece of meat or some other food stuck in your esophagus, you may choose to ride it out if it's not interfering with your breathing and you're still able to swallow. The food will plop down into the stomach within a few hours. A few sips of water or a cup of gelatin, yogurt, or some other semi-solid food will stimulate the swallowing reflex and help to push the food down into the stomach.

If you are drooling, and your chest feels as though you swallowed a keg of nails, you need to get to a hospital right away. This is a dangerous situation. An obstructed esophagus may perforate, and you might aspirate food and saliva into your lungs. If nothing else, you will become dehydrated from lack of water.

Adolph's meat tenderizer is a traditional remedy for food caught in the esophagus. There's no doubt that it works. Problem is, it can burn a hole in your esophagus. Save it for the roast.

Fish and chicken bones can get hung up in the upper esophagus. They are not big enough to obstruct the airway, but they can make swallowing a real pain. Have your buddy shine a bright light into the back of your throat. He should be able to see the bone overlying one of the tonsils and remove it with needle-nose pliers or a Q-tip.

Here are some tips to keep you from biting off more than you can chew:

1. Cut your food into small pieces and chew slowly.
2. Don't laugh and talk while you're chewing.
3. Ease up on the alcohol before and during meals.

8

HYPOTHERMIA

"A certain fear of death, dull and oppressive, came to him. This fear quickly became poignant as he realized that it was no longer a matter of freezing his fingers and toes, or of losing his hands and feet, but that it was a matter of life and death with the chances against him. This threw him into a panic, and he turned and ran up the creek bed along the old, dim trail. He ran blindly, without intention, in such fear as he had never known in his life. . . . Without doubt, he would lose some fingers and toes and some of his face; but the boys would take care of him, and save the rest of him when he got there. And at the same time there was another thought in his mind that said he would never get to the camp . . . that it was too many miles away, that the freezing had too great a start on him, and that he would soon be stiff and dead."

—JACK LONDON,
"To Build a Fire"

છે

A few years ago, during the spring salmon run on Lake George, a man capsized his small aluminum boat while trying to land a large fish. He was in the frigid water for an hour before he was rescued. It appeared that he was going to do all right when he climbed on deck and went below to warm up. He collapsed in the cabin and died of hypothermia.

Cold is a relentless enemy. You don't really defeat it; you survive it. If you're lucky. It cannot be denied, only stalled. If you're exposed to it long enough, it will beat you. Probing with icy fingers, it finds a chink in your armor, and exploits the breach in your defenses until it has sucked the warmth out of your marrow, dooming you to the fate of the man in Jack London's classic story.

71

Whether you are bobbing in the chilly waters of Lake George or stranded in a snowstorm on a Rocky Mountain peak, your body will be under siege from the cold. It will mount a feverish struggle to preserve warmth, but once your core temperature drops below 95 degrees F, you're hypothermic. Then you are on a slippery slope, and it's only a matter of time before your body's caloric reserve is depleted, your internal organs shut down, and your heart stops beating.

Mechanisms of Heat Loss

Actually, there isn't any such thing as "cold." What we perceive as cold is merely the absence of heat. But it is convenient to think of cold as a kind of magnet that pulls the heat out of your body through the following mechanisms:

1. *Conduction.* The direct transfer of heat from the body to a cooler object. Normally not a major mechanism of heat loss, it is *the* major cause of heat loss during cold water immersion.
2. *Convection.* The loss of heat by circulation of the air or liquid in which the body is immersed. Movement of the medium breaks up the thin layer of warm particles on the surface of the body. A fan cools by convection, and "wind chill" plays a big role in cooling on windy days.
3. *Radiation.* The loss of heat through emitted energy. It normally accounts for over half of the body's heat loss.
4. *Evaporation.* Heat lost when sweat or water on the body's surface is changed into steam. For each gram of water that evaporates from the skin, 580 calories of heat are lost. Perspiration increases evaporative heat loss, as does wet clothing on a windy day.

Rising to the Challenge

Humans are warm-blooded animals. We keep our internal temperature right around 98.6 degrees F. We even have a thermostat, a part of the brain called the "thermoregulatory center." When "cold" signals arrive from the millions of thermal sensors in the skin and elsewhere in the body, the thermostat, acting through the sympathetic nervous system (see Chapter 1), does a number of things to increase heat production and decrease heat loss:

1. The muscles start to shiver, increasing heat production fivefold. Vigorous exercise increases heat production by 1,000 percent.

2. Blood vessels in the skin and limbs constrict. This limits radiant heat loss from the body surface, but even more important, it preserves the flow of warm blood to a core of vital organs (brain, heart, lungs, and digestive organs) and shunts blood from the cold shell of skin, muscle, and fat—sort of like the pioneers drawing their wagons up in a circle to defend themselves against the Indians.

3. The heart beats faster and harder.

4. Sweating stops, decreasing evaporative heat loss.

5. The metabolic rate increases up to sixfold, increasing the heat generated by the chemical reactions in each cell.

That Slippery Slope

The body's furious response to the cold is like turning on your car heater when you're stranded somewhere. It's great while it lasts, but sooner or later you're going to run out of gas. When that happens, the situation deteriorates in a hurry. Eventually, the muscles become too tired and too energy-starved to shiver. They become stiff and sluggish when the core temperature drops below 90 degrees. And the heart and metabolism slow, fluid shifts out of the circulation into the spaces between the cells, fluid is lost through the kidneys, and the blood pressure drops. With further cooling, the brain becomes sluggish, and the heart becomes irritable. Below 80 degrees, you become stiff and unresponsive, and have no detectable pulses. You may mistakenly be declared dead.

Predisposing Causes

Here are some things that can help to turn you into Frosty the Snowman:

1. *Exposure to the elements.* You can become hypothermic in the Yukon Territory just about any day, and you can become hypothermic in Georgia or anywhere else when the conditions are right. That means cool temperatures (not necessarily below freezing), high wind, and low humidity.

2. *Cold-water immersion.* Water is a much greater heat conductor than air, and you'll cool at least 100 times faster in water than in air at the same temperature. This effect is compounded by movement and exposure of areas of high heat loss, such as the head, neck, and face.

3. *Immobility.* A fracture or other disabling injury is a double whammy: not only does it interfere with one of your first lines of defense against hypo-

thermia (increased muscle activity and shivering), it also makes it harder for you to get out of the cold.

4. *Drugs and alcohol.* Alcohol and cold are compatible—if you are a lizard. Lizards and other cold-blooded creatures don't have to worry about a thermostat. They just go with the flow. Alcohol screws up the thermostat, inhibits shivering, impairs judgment, and dilates the blood vessels in the skin. Those Saint Bernard dogs they used to send out with the whiskey barrel around their necks always came back alone.

How to Recognize Hypothermia

To diagnose hypothermia, you have to think of it. If your buddy has been buried under an avalanche, you are going to be thinking about it. If he's been sitting out in the bay in a duck boat on a cold, blustery day, you may not. But you should always be thinking "hypothermia" whenever one of the predisposing factors is in play.

The most reliable sign of *mild hypothermia* (core temperature 90 to 95 degrees) is shivering. But you must be sensitive to some of the more subtle signs, such as thick or slurred speech, confusion, difficulty keeping up with the group, and incoordination. The victim of mild hypothermia may have trouble zipping his fly or hammering tent stakes into the ground, and his skin may be cool to the touch.

The guy who had been shivering, but has stopped, and now is confused and indifferent to his surroundings, has *severe hypothermia.* His core temperature is below 90 degrees, and his skin is cold to the touch, and pale or blue and mottled. His pulse may be weak, slow, and irregular. He's forgetful, and neglects to cover up from the cold, leaving his jacket unzipped and his mittens and hat off. He may even undress or make other dangerous errors in judgment. His clothing may be soaked with urine, and he may have the fruity smell of acetone on his breath, a sign of disrupted metabolism.

Treatment of Hypothermia

When a guy is drowning, you get him out of the water first, and then worry about resuscitating him. It's the same story with hypothermia. The first order of business is to get the victim out of the cold and wind, remove any wet clothing, and take measures to limit further heat loss. Cover up his head and neck, and make sure he's not in contact with the cold ground.

The next priority is to decide whether you are dealing with mild or severe hypothermia. (This is not an academic distinction. If you try rewarming the victim of severe hypothermia in the field, you may kill him.)

If he is suffering from *mild hypothermia,* give him dry clothing and have him crawl inside a sleeping bag, either alone or with someone else. Or you can throw a blanket around him and let him sit by the fire. Hot toddies are out, but you can give him a cup of hot cocoa or cider.

The victim of *severe hypothermia* has to be handled the same way you'd handle an angry porcupine: *very* gently. The heart becomes irritable when it's cold. Physical exertion can cause cold, acidic blood in the cold shell to surge into the heart, causing it to fibrillate. Don't let him get up or move around. Gently place him in a sleeping bag or under a blanket with one or two other people while you arrange for medical evacuation.

If evacuation isn't feasible, you will have to rewarm him in the field, using the radiant heat from a fire, chemical "hot packs," hot-water bottles, or warmed stones or other objects. Hot baths are *verboten.* They cause the blood vessels in the skin and extremities to dilate and fill with warm blood from the core. The blood volume is already compromised by loss of fluid into the tissues and from the kidneys, so this leads to "rewarming shock." And when the now-cold blood returns to the heart, it can cause a temperature "afterdrop" and fibrillation.

CPR and Hypothermia

The victim of hypothermia may be stiff, unresponsive, and pale, and may have fixed and dilated pupils. But he is not dead until he is warm and dead. Do CPR unless he has a lethal injury, his chest is frozen, he is breathing or moving, or doing CPR would put his rescuers in danger.

You may elect *not* to do CPR if his core temperature is below 28 degrees centigrade (82.4 degrees F) and equal to the ambient temperature, he's been immersed in water for more than 50 minutes, or you are more than four hours from a hospital.

?❧ PREVENTING HYPOTHERMIA: DRESS FOR SUCCESS

Your body may be a temple, but it is also a heat-generating machine. If you are physically fit, you will be able to maintain your body heat longer on the trail, and you'll have a better chance of getting to shelter if the weather turns nasty. Get yourself into shape with good aerobic and muscle conditioning before you answer the call of the wild in winter.

Drink plenty of fluids when you are outside in the cold. Your metabolic furnace cannot run at full capacity if you are dehydrated. And dehydration increases the risk of frostbite.

You should also keep that metabolic furnace stoked with plenty of calories, especially the carbohydrate variety. And make sure you bring some snacks along with you on the trail.

When it comes to hypothermia, clothes make the man. Exercise is great, but jumping jacks alone aren't going to do it. Clothing can dramatically decrease conductive and convective heat losses. Air is a great insulator, so the key is to maintain multiple layers of warm air around your body. And the way to do that is by wearing multiple layers of clothing, which you can shed or add to as weather conditions change. The last thing you want to do is to sweat excessively. That accelerates evaporative heat loss. You can doff hat and gloves when you start to feel warm, and then loosen up your collar or take off your jacket and one or two underlayers as conditions dictate.

The best cold-weather materials are wool (which retains its insulating properties when wet), down, foam, Orlon, Dacron, polyester, Gore-Tex, Thinsulate, taslanized nylon, and Flectalon. Cotton wets easily, and its "wicking" action causes rapid cooling. You'd survive longer stark naked than in wet cotton in the cold.

Your cold-weather wardrobe might look something like this: wool underwear (polypropylene, Capilene or Olefin is a good choice if you anticipate working up a sweat), wool pants and shirts, wool sweater, a jacket or vest filled with down, Quallofil or some other lofting material and having a two-way zipper, a hooded nylon or Gore-Tex parka or windbreaker, windproof and water-repellent wind pants, two pair of socks (polypropylene and wool), a wool stocking cap or balaclava, wool or wool-lined polypropylene mittens with nylon or Gore-Tex shells, and rubber-soled, leather climbing boots or double winter mountaineering boots. Select boots with thick soles and insoles to impede conductive heat loss through the feet, and plenty of toe room. Tight boots cut off the circulation to the toes and leave no room for a layer of insulating air between sock and uppers.

≥◦ IMMERSION HYPOTHERMIA

Cold water is a relentless killer. It knifes through your clothing, overwhelms the insulating capacity of your subcutaneous fat, and sucks the warmth out of your very core. And water doesn't have to have ice floes in it to qualify as "cold water." You can become hypothermic in 77-degree water. Most American coastal waters and lakes are cooler than that *year round,* even the waters of Honolulu and San Diego.

There is a common misconception that falling into frigid water is tantamount to instant death. Actually, that's rare. When it happens, it's because the gasp reflex causes you to inhale water and drown. The fact is, you can survive for several hours in 50- to 60-degree water, depending on your body type and other factors. The body's core temperature remains stable for 15 minutes in cold water. Time enough to save yourself, if you know what to do.

What happens when you fall into cold water:

1. The cold water on your skin stimulates the respiratory center in the brain, causing you to gasp and then hyperventilate for a minute or two. All that respiratory stimulation diminishes your breath-holding capacity to 15 to 25 seconds. Not good if you're trapped underwater.
2. The blood vessels in your skin and muscles constrict, shutting off blood flow to the periphery and forming that cold "shell" insulating a warm "core." Your skin turns blue, you break out in goose bumps, and your movements become sluggish, making it harder for you to pull yourself out of the water. Fine motor tasks, such as operating a boat radio and using signaling devices, become impossible.
3. You begin to shiver. Shivering is the body's main defense against hypothermia in air, but in water it's a mixed blessing. It increases metabolic heat production by 500 percent, but it also increases the flow of water between skin and clothing, accelerating convective heat loss (the "flushing effect").
4. As your core temperature drops below 90 degrees, you stop shivering and you start to get a little wacky. You become confused, your judgment becomes impaired, and you may even hallucinate. Immersion victims have been known to remove their personal flotation devices (PFDs) and clothing, or attempt to swim for shore, even when shore is not in sight.

Because of its greater thermal conductivity and specific heat, you cool 100 times faster in water than in air at the same temperature. The head and extremities cool most rapidly, because of their greater surface to volume ratio, but heat loss from the trunk is more critical to survival. Heat escapes quickly from the groin and neck, where blood passes through large vessels immediately under the skin surface.

Not everyone who goes into the drink cools at the same rate. How fast a person cools depends on several factors:

1. *Body fat.* This is *the* most important factor. Eskimos know what an excellent insulator blubber is. The fatter you are, the slower you cool in water.

2. *Body type.* Big people cool slower than smaller people, and kids cool faster than adults. Women have more fat, but are usually smaller, so they cool at the same rate as men.

3. *Physical fitness.* A double-edged sword. Cardiovascular fitness may help you to handle the stress of cold water immersion, but this benefit is outweighed by the fact that fit people have less subcutaneous fat for insulation. So the fat and unfit probably have at least as good a shot at surviving immersion as the iron man triathlete.

4. *Water temperature.* The colder the water, the faster you cool.

5. *Clothing.* Conventional thermal clothing, designed to take advantage of the insulating effect of pockets of air trapped between skin and garment, is of little value in water. These air pockets are history as soon as you hit the drink. But protective clothing has been developed that minimizes the loss of trapped air.

"Wet" garments trap air in bubbles in tight-fitted wet suits or in loose-fitted coveralls or flotation jackets. Insulated coveralls are a good choice for recreational fishermen. They have nylon covers, closed-cell foam insulation, foam neoprene hoods, reflective tape, 29 to 38 pounds of buoyancy, and fit like snowmobile suits. They are easy to put on, don't hinder movement, and provide protection from cold air as well as cold water.

"Dry" garments (survival suits) have watertight wrist, ankle, and neck seals that keep covered areas dry. They provide twice the insulation of insulated coveralls, and their effectiveness isn't diminished in rough seas. (The cooling rate in "wet" garments nearly doubles in rough water, due to the "flushing effect.") They are cumbersome, however, and not practical for recreational fishermen.

6. *Alcohol.* If you are drunk, you are more apt to fall off a dock or out of a boat. In that case, you're more likely to drown than die of hypothermia. And while alcohol doesn't significantly increase your cooling rate in water, it may impair your judgment and coordination to the point that you can't do the things you need to do to save yourself.

7. *Behavior.* Swimming and treading water increase the flow of warm blood from the body's core to the muscles, breaking down the "shell" insulation and increasing the cooling rate 35 to 50 percent. Exercise also accelerates cooling by increasing the flow of cold water under protective clothing. If you are wearing a PFD, you won't have to tread water or swim.

If you go into the drink, stay with the boat, and get out of the water if you can. At least pull yourself as far out of the water as possible. Try to conserve energy and body heat, and exercise as little as possible. Avoid the open body position in the water, cover the sides of the chest and groin, and go into the Heat Escape Lessening Posture (HELP) (see Figure 15). A group of people should huddle in a tight circle, with children in the center. Remember, 75 percent of heat loss is from the head; cover it and keep it clear of the water.

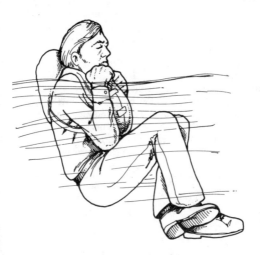

15. The HELP position.

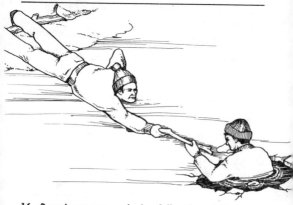

16. *Rescuing someone who has fallen through the ice.*

(The best way to rescue a person who has fallen through the ice is to assume the prone position and reach out to him with a stick. Keep your feet anchored onshore so that you aren't pulled into the water.)

When the rescue boat pulls up and plucks you from the lake, you may be out of the water, but you're still not out of the woods. The fisherman who collapsed after being pulled out of Lake George died of vascular collapse. Walking or any other physical exercise, jarring movements, rewarming shock, and core temperature "afterdrop" can all cause sudden death. That's what happened to the salmon fisherman on the rescue boat.

The cold water immersion victim has to be handled very carefully. *Move him as little as possible.* Keep him horizontal, do CPR if necessary, and keep him from getting any colder by *gently* removing wet clothing, drying his skin, and keeping him out of the wind. Then apply hot packs to the neck, sides of the chest, and groin. Or take your clothes off and get into a sleeping bag or under some blankets with him. A hot bath or shower is fine for moderate hypothermia. If he has severe hypothermia, arrange for medical evacuation.

FROSTBITE AND OTHER COLD INJURIES

During its disastrous invasion of Russia in 1812, Napoleon's Grande Armée was devastated by cold injury. This was due in no small part to the fact that soldiers with frostbite spent their nights thawing their frozen limbs over roaring fires, only to refreeze them the next day.

On the Eastern Front in World War II, the winter of 1941–42 was the coldest in over a century. The Russians, with the help of their two greatest commanders, "General January" and "General February," dashed Hitler's hopes for a quick victory over the Soviet Union by repelling the Nazi invaders on the outskirts of Moscow. German casualties from frostbite numbered 112,627.

A few winters ago, a fisherman froze his feet while ice fishing on a lake in Minnesota. He built a fire and thawed them out, then refroze them while hiking back to his car that evening. He eventually lost eight toes.

Whether you wage your winter campaigns on the Russian steppes or on ice-covered lakes in Alaska or Minnesota, your real enemy is frostbite. This is one foe you don't want to underestimate. It'll sneak up and nibble at your fingers and toes, turning them into so many links of frozen sausage. But you can turn the tables on the cold and nip frostbite in the bud, if you know its modus operandi.

Predisposing Factors

Frostbite is tissue injury or death caused by exposure to subfreezing cold. Predisposing factors include

1. *Ambient temperature.* Frostbite is more likely to occur in temperatures below 20 degrees F.
2. *Wind chill.* A cold wind whipping across your face will take the color out of your cheeks in no

time, as convection accelerates the cooling process. Tissues don't become cooler than ambient temperature, but they cool faster.

3. *High altitude.* Because it's colder up there, mainly. But the thinner air also seems to aggravate cold injury, and the storms are more violent.

4. *Alcohol and drugs.* You won't know enough to come in out of the cold, or pull on a hat and mittens, if you're sloshed. You're also more likely to fall and break an arm or leg, increasing your risk of hypothermia *and* frostbite.

5. *Conduction injury.* You remember that old story about not touching cold metal with exposed flesh—how your finger or tongue would freeze to the metal. It's true. Metal and most other materials are much better heat conductors than air. On a cold day, a sled runner or the barrel of a gun extracts heat from your hand the way a magnet attracts iron filings. So does water. The freezing point of gasoline and other volatile hydrocarbons is lower than that of water; it's minus 70 degrees F. Spill some on your hand on a cold day and it's instant frostbite.

6. *Fatigue.* Vince Lombardi said, "Fatigue makes cowards of us all." It also makes us candidates for hypothermia and frostbite by depleting our energy reserves.

7. *Underlying illness.* Diabetes and circulatory disorders impair the circulation to the extremities, setting the stage for frostbite.

8. *Tobacco.* Nicotine puts the vise-grip on the small arteries in the skin and extremities, opening the door for cold injury.

9. *Previous frostbite.* Once you've been initiated into the Frostbite Club, you're a lifetime member, and always vulnerable to repeat cold injury.

10. *Deep snow.* Standing or walking in deep, loose snow will cool your piggies real quick. It is much colder deep down in the snow than on the surface.

Mechanism of Injury

Here's what happened to the ice fisherman in Minnesota. After sitting out in the open on a frozen lake for several hours, he became mildly hypothermic. The blood vessels in his skin and extremities clamped down in order to minimize further heat loss. The ice he was standing on drew the warmth out of his feet, and the skin and subcutaneous tissues of his toes froze. Chilled arterioles just beneath the frozen tissues reflexively constricted, the blood in the capillaries became more viscous, and the flow of blood through these capillaries slowed nearly to a halt. The blood became thick and syrupy and clots formed, blocking the capillary bed and depriving the tissues of badly needed oxygen and nutrients. Shunts running from arterioles to venules then diverted blood away from the capillary beds. These shunts opened and closed in cycles, like the valves on a steam pipe, allowing waves of warm blood to surge into the feet from time to time. When the fisherman's core temperature dropped farther, these shunts stayed open for good, and the tissues began to freeze.

As the tissues cooled, ice crystals formed in the spaces outside the cells. These crystals then pulled water out of the cells, dehydrating them, disrupting their cell membranes, and throwing a monkey wrench into their metabolic machinery.

The original frostbite injury to the fisherman's toes was severe enough. His tootsies got the knock-out punch when they were refrozen on the hike back to his car. I hope he at least caught some fish.

Signs and Symptoms

Because of their distance from the warm core, and because of their large surface-to-volume ratio, which predisposes to more rapid cooling, the feet, hands, ears, and nose are most vulnerable to frostbite. There have been reports of frostbite to the penis in joggers, but we can only speculate whether that is attributable to the part's distance from the core or an unusually high surface-to-volume ratio.

The first response to cold is usually a stinging pain, followed by numbness and blanching of the tissue. This is known as *frostnip*. It looks like a small white patch on the cheeks, nose or ears. Frostnip is easily treated by immediate rewarming.

Frostnip that is ignored progresses to *superficial frostbite*. This involves frozen skin and subcutaneous tissues. The skin remains bloodless, pale or gray, and cool to the touch. The tissue beneath the surface remains soft and pliable. A day or so after the injury, large blisters pop up like mushrooms. After a few days, the blisters heal, and a hard, dry *eschar* forms. This is a thick, black scar that separates from the underlying tissue in a few weeks, and is replaced by new, red skin which eventually takes on a normal appearance.

Deep frostbite implies freezing of superficial as

well as deep structures, including nerve, muscle, tendon, and even bone. The part is purple or red, cool to the touch, and anesthetic. The limb is as hard as a piece of wood. In contrast to superficial frostbite, in which the injured part is sensitive, warm, and pink after rewarming, the part remains cold and blue after thawing. Small blood blisters may form after 1 to 3 weeks, and the part may remain swollen for months after. Eventually it will mummify and fall off.

Treatment

You can treat frostnipped hands anywhere, anytime, by breathing through cupped hands or by putting your hands in your armpits. But there's a time and place for treatment of frostbite. The place is *indoors* and the time is when you are sure there is no chance that the thawed part will be refrozen. Avoid the freeze-thaw-refreeze cycle at all costs. It is infinitely better to walk out of the wilderness on frostbitten feet than to thaw them out and risk the chance of their refreezing later. Before you start out for the warming hut, first remove and replace all wet clothing and tight boots. And stay away from campfires and car heaters and mufflers en route.

Start thawing the injured part as soon as you get to a secure shelter. The key to recovery from frostbite is *rapid rewarming*. Fill a large container with water heated to between 104–108 degrees F (40–42 degrees C), and immerse the part in it. Make sure that you remove all jewelry and constrictive clothing, and don't allow the part to rest on the bottom or sides of the vessel.

That frozen foot or hand will cool the bath like a block of ice, so you'll have to add warm water at frequent intervals. Ensure against scalding insensitive tissues by never using water warmer than an uninjured hand can tolerate and by thoroughly stirring the water before reimmersing the limb.

Rewarm until the skin becomes soft and flushed. This should take no more than 30 minutes. And don't forget to warm the whole person! There is no point in rewarming a frozen foot if the circulation to the foot is still shut down due to hypothermia.

After the Ice-out

When you are done rewarming the limb, gently dry it with a clean towel, then elevate it on a pillow and fashion a protective cradle to keep blankets off it. Place sterile gauze or cotton between the digits to absorb moisture, and apply aloe vera or triple antibiotic ointment to the damaged skin. Then elevate the injured part on a pillow and leave it open to the air.

Bathe the frostbitten part in a warm bath with mild soap twice a day. This cleans the debris from the wounds, reduces the chance of infection, and stimulates the circulation. It's also a good time to do gentle, active range-of-motion exercises to prevent stiffness in the digits. But try to resist that primitive human urge to pop the blisters. They will go away on their own bye and bye.

One or two aspirins or ibuprofens twice a day may improve microcirculation and enhance healing. A few extra glasses of water or fruit juice each day will aid in rehydrating the frostbite/hypothermia victim and give the circulation a big boost.

Prevention of Frostbite

A few words to the wise:

1. Eat mountains of nutritious foods in cold weather to keep that metabolic furnace stoked. (You'll get more bang for the buck from fats at low altitude.)
2. Don't set out on a long trek too early in the morning, or when the weather threatens to turn nasty.
3. Tight boots have caused more cases of frostbite than the arctic express. Shun constrictive clothing, plastic boots, and tight crampon straps.
4. Dress for success. Keep your head, neck, and face covered. On extremely cold days, tie a cloth over your face below your eyes and let it hang loosely. It will allow you to breathe and yet keep your face warm. Wear mittens instead of gloves, and keep them attached to the end of a string draped around your neck. Keep your socks dry and wrinkle-free. Always bring along extra socks and mittens. You can stick a few feathers or some dry grass or moss inside your shoes for extra insulation.
5. Wash your hands, face, and feet sparingly in cold weather. Soap and water remove protective oils; shaving removes the layer of dead cells that protects against the wind and cold. You want skin like a shark's in rough weather.
6. Never touch metal with your bare hands in cold weather. Metal parts that must be touched with the bare hands should be wrapped with adhesive tape.
7. Keep your fingernails and toenails trimmed.

8. Allow several hours to recover from mild hypothermia.
9. Treat alcohol and tobacco as though they were bad for you.
10. No matter what happens out there, don't panic. Remember, sweat accelerates evaporation and heat loss.

?✺ OTHER COLD INJURIES

Trench Foot (Immersion Foot)

So-called because it was a common injury during the trench warfare of World War I. It is caused by vasoconstriction secondary to prolonged standing or walking in cold water. After sloshing around in cold puddles for a few hours or days, the feet become cold, pale, waxy, pulseless, and numb. Upon rewarming, blood flow returns with a vengeance, and the foot becomes hot, red, and swollen. Not to mention painful. The swelling eventually subsides, but the foot remains weak, sweaty, and sensitive to the cold for years.

Prevention of trench foot is simply a matter of avoiding prolonged walking or standing in marshes, bogs, and stream beds, and avoiding tight boots or shoes.

Treatment consists of simply removing wet boots and socks and rewarming the feet with warm blankets or by resting them in a buddy's armpits. Avoid weight-bearing for a day or so after the feet are rewarmed.

Chilblains (Pernio)

When I think of chilblains, I think of one of those nineteenth-century English novels, like *Great Expectations* or *Wuthering Heights,* where someone is always running across the moor, exposing his skin to the wet and wind. When the arms, shins, knees, hands, or cheeks are exposed to raw, wet weather (such as prevails in England and northern Europe), the skin becomes red, itchy, warm, tender, and swollen. Chronic exposure to such weather conditions can produce skin that is red, rough, and cool to the touch.

Warm protective clothing protects the skin from chilblains. A bland moisturizing ointment is as good treatment as any.

10

SOLAR INJURIES AND HEAT ILLNESS

"Mad dogs and Englishmen go out in the midday sun."

—NOEL COWARD

∂∾

Chicken Little was right. Sort of. The sky isn't exactly falling, but it has sprung a leak. There's a big hole in the ozone layer over the South Pole, and it's getting threadbare everywhere else. All those chlorofluorocarbons, atmospheric pollutants, and jet aircraft are destroying ozone molecules. The less ozone there is up there in the ozonosphere, the more destructive ultraviolet radiation (UVR) strikes the earth's surface. And that's bad news for mad dogs, Englishmen, and outdoor sportsmen.

∂∾ THE ELECTROMAGNETIC SPECTRUM

The sun's rays contain a broad spectrum of electromagnetic radiation, ranging from cosmic rays to radio waves. Two thirds of this radiation is absorbed, scattered, or reflected by the atmosphere. Ozone absorbs UVR with wavelengths in the range 220–290 nanometers (UVC). But significant amounts of ultraviolet B (UVB, 290–320 nm wavelength) and ultraviolet A (UVA, wavelength 320–400) penetrate the atmosphere. UVB causes sunburn, tanning, premature aging, and skin cancer. UVA is responsible for "sun cataracts" and sun allergies.

Sunlight is like cholesterol. A little bit is not only good for you but essential for life. In fact, UVB converts a form of cholesterol into vitamin D in the skin.

longer wavelength →		higher energy →
	Cosmic rays	
	Gamma rays	
	X-rays	
	Vacuum ultraviolet	
	UVC	
	UVB	
	UVA	
	Visible light	
	Infrared	
	Microwaves	
	Radio waves	

?☞ HOW MUCH SUN CAN YOU HANDLE?

How much UVR you can take before your skin turns to burned leather depends on a number of factors. The most important of these is your skin type. Whether you tan or burn depends on the number of pigment particles (melanosomes) in the pigment-producing cells (melanocytes) in your epidermis. And that is genetically determined. Melanocytes produce *melanin,* the dark pigment that causes tanning and blocks transmission of UVB into the deeper layers of the skin. Blonds and redheads with blue or green eyes have relatively few melanocytes, burn easily, and almost never tan.

Skin Type	Burning/Tanning Characteristics	Examples
I	always burns, never tans	blonds and redheads, blue eyes
II	Usually burns, tans after many hours in the sun	fair skinned, blonds
III	burns and tans moderately	most Caucasians
IV	burns slightly, tans well	Hispanics and Asians
V	almost never burns, tans darkly	Middle Easterners, Indians
VI	burns only with very heavy exposure	Blacks

✍ DETERMINANTS OF UVR INTENSITY

You are stuck with the skin you were born with, but you do have control over some of the other factors that determine your exposure to UVR. It helps to be familiar with the "solar zenith angle." This is the angle at which the rays strike the earth's surface. The sharper the angle, the greater distance they have to travel through the atmosphere, and the more UVR is absorbed. The solar zenith angle, in turn, is a function of the *time of day, time of year,* and *latitude*.

Do you remember how the sheriff (Gary Cooper) couldn't get anyone to come outside and help him fight the bad guys in the movie *High Noon?* Those people weren't afraid of the gun slingers. They just didn't want to get roasted in the noonday sun. The sun is most directly overhead at noon. Sunlight passes through the atmosphere most directly then, so less UVR is absorbed. You can get deep fried between the hours of 9 A.M. and 3 P.M. That's when 80 percent of the UVB for the day strikes the earth's surface. (UVA intensity, on the other hand, remains almost constant throughout the day.) And sunlight is most intense during the summer months, when the sun traverses a more northerly (or southerly, if you live in the southern hemisphere) route in the sky. Your UVR exposure per unit time is much less on a sunny winter day than on a summer day. If you are smart, you will apportion more of your outdoor activities to the winter months.

The third determinant of the solar zenith angle is latitude. The sun's rays strike the earth perpendicularly at the equator and more obliquely with increasing latitude. The solar zenith angle and intensity of solar radiation decrease as you travel farther north or south of the equator. So, if you've got a choice between tarpon fishing in the Florida Keys or trout fishing in Ontario, head north.

Altitude has a lot to do with the amount of UVR to which you are exposed. The atmosphere is thinner at higher altitudes, and there are less water vapor, smoke, and dust to filter UVR. Figure on 4 to 5 percent more UVR for each 1,000 feet of elevation. Keep that in mind when you plan your next backpacking trip to the high mountain lakes for golden trout. And glaciers and snowfields reflect 85 percent of the ultraviolet radiation that strikes their surfaces, adding to the already considerable direct light. Elk hunters beware!

Atmospheric conditions affect the intensity of UVR. Smoke absorbs UVR. Dust and water scatter it. I learned this firsthand when I was out in Wyoming in 1988. The fires in nearby Yellowstone were still raging, and a dense smoke cloud hung in the air, almost blotting out the sun. I have skin type I, yet I didn't get a hint of sunburn, despite being out in the midday sun every day. On the other hand, UVR penetrates the densest cloud cover, while heat-carrying infrared waves are filtered out. That makes cool, overcast days dangerous. Because it's not warm and "sunny" out, you don't appreciate the intensity of the sun's rays and fail to cover up. And you can't hide in the shade on hazy days; the sun's rays are "bent" by the haze and reflected into shady areas.

Wind and sun are a potent combination. Together they cause "windburn." Wind drys the skin, removing urocanic acid, a natural skin protector, and irritates sunburned skin.

Even fishermen with skin types III and IV will be sunburned after a day out on the water. That's because sunlight bounces off the water's surface and into your face. This is called *reflectivity*. Substances have different reflectivities. Water is 100 percent reflective at noon, but only 10 percent reflective in the early morning and evening. (Choppy water is much more reflective than calm water.) Snow is highly reflective (85 percent), while sand has a reflectivity of 20 percent, and grass 2.5 percent. You'll get less UVR hunting jackrabbits in the high desert in the winter than hunting snowshoe hares on a snowfield at the same elevation and latitude.

≈ PHOTOSENSITIVITY REACTIONS

UVR can get to you in many different ways. It can combine with certain chemicals, known as *photosensitizers,* to cause an exaggerated response to sunlight. Photosensitivity reactions can take the form of a severe sunburn (phototoxicity) or an allergic reaction resulting in an eczemalike rash (photoallergy). A burn that continues to worsen over a period of days is probably a phototoxic reaction. They are caused by both UVA and UVB radiation and are quite common. Photoallergic reactions are triggered by UVA radiation and are uncommon.

A partial list of photosensitizers includes food additives (cyclamates and saccharine), shaving creams and aftershave lotions, sulfa antibiotics, certain antihistamines and tranquilizers, oral diabetes medications and diuretics, tetracycline antibiotics, benzocaine (used in most spray anesthetics), barbiturates, bithionol (used in soaps and first aid creams), green soap, some sunscreens, and certain plants.

A twist of lemon can brighten your drink. Skin contact with lemon, lime, parsley, celery, parsnip, fig, carrot and other plants, followed by a dash of UVR, can light up your skin in a type of photosensitivity reaction called *phytophotodermatitis*. You may get a fierce sunburn or (rarely) an allergic rash resembling poison ivy.

?❧ SKIN CANCER

Skin cancer is a recreational hazard for hunters and fishermen. "The sun is the cause of at least 90 percent of skin cancers," according to the Skin Cancer Foundation. They predict a worldwide epidemic of skin cancer in the coming years if the current growth rate continues. They also predict that "during the next decade, 5 million men and women in the United States will learn that they have skin cancer ... 90 percent of those cancers will appear on the face and other exposed parts of the body. Hundreds of thousands will be disfigured through the total or partial loss of noses ... eyes ... lips ... ears ... 50,000 will die of the disease or its complications."

Basal cell carcinoma, the most common skin cancer, is a painless, smooth, waxy thickening of the skin. It's easy to ignore. It grows very slowly, but it will bore straight down through the skin, muscle, fat, and even bone. It can kill you if you let it.

Look at the tops of your hands. Now examine your face in a mirror. Do you see any scaly, rough thickenings, white things that you've picked at that won't go away? These may be *solar keratoses,* the product of chronic exposure to the sun. They won't hurt you, usually. But every once in a while, a solar keratosis turns into a *squamous cell carcinoma.* These are painless, red nodules with scales. They are highly curable if they are removed before they spread to other parts of the body.

Malignant melanoma, the deadly "black mole," was a rare cancer 50 years ago. It now strikes over 23,000 Americans each year, and by the year 2000, 1 out of every 100 Americans can expect to be diagnosed with malignant melanoma at some time in their lives. Skin types I and II are especially vulnerable to melanoma. Early detection is the only hope for a cure.

The only sure way to avoid sunburn and sun-damaged skin is to join the submarine service. But there are a few things that you can do short of that.

- *Limit your exposure.* Time your forays into the outdoors carefully. Stay in the shade during the hours of maximum sun intensity, 9 A.M. to 3 P.M.
- *Wear protective clothing.* Tight-mesh clothing blocks nearly all UVR when dry. Wet or loose mesh clothing transmits a significant amount of UVR. Wear a long-sleeved shirt and long pants, and a broad-brimmed hat or a baseball hat with a "Foreign Legion" flap in the back to protect your neck.
- *Use sunscreens and sunblockers.* Sunscreens are creams, gels, oils, or lotions containing chemicals that absorb ultraviolet radiation. They can help to prevent sunburn, photosensitivity reactions, and skin cancer. Since sunburn is caused by UVB, and most photosensitivity reactions are triggered by UVA, you should choose a sunscreen containing either benzophenone or anthranilate, chemicals that absorb both UVA and UVB.

Sunscreens are rated according to their sun protection factor (SPF). If you are wearing a sunscreen with an SPF of 5, you could, theoretically, stay out in the sun five times longer before burning than you could if your skin was unprotected. If your skin burns moderately, you should use a sunscreen with an SPF of 6 to 8. If you have fair skin, you should use a sunscreen with an SPF of at least 15. Liberally apply the sunscreen to all exposed skin 30 minutes to 1 hour prior to exposure so that it can penetrate to the deep layers. And reapply it after swimming or sweating, even if you are using a "waterproof" brand. (*Warning:* Reapplying sunscreen doesn't extend the total time that you can spend in the sun.)

Many of the chemicals used in sunscreens, including cinnamates, oxybenzone, and para-aminobenzoic acid (PABA), can cause rashes and photosensitivity reactions. If you are sensitive to these chemicals, you can use physical sunblocks. These are opaque creams or pastes that block transmission of all types of solar radiation. Examples of physical sunblocks include talc, zinc oxide, titanium oxide, kaolin, red veterinary petrolatum, and red ferric oxide. Dab a little on areas that are especially likely to burn, such as your nose, ears, cheeks, lips, and neck. If you are caught out in the sun without a sunscreen, try axle grease, charcoal or wood ashes, or a paste of clay. If you are at the seashore, you can make "sunburn powder" of lime. Burn seashells or coral over an open fire and pulverize them into a powder. Then, make a paste by mixing the powder with oil or water, and apply it over all exposed skin. Or expose coconut meat to the sun to make a coconut oil sunscreen.

〰 TREATMENT OF SUNBURN

There's nothing new under the sun in the treatment of sunburn. Cool compresses with milk and water or Burow's solution, or just lying in a cool stream, can provide merciful, if temporary, relief from the pain of sunburn. Noxzema, Cetaphil, and other soothing lotions and creams help, and aspirin, acetaminophen, or ibuprofen can be counted on to take the edge off the sting.

Anesthetic sprays offer short-term relief at best, and usually contain benzocaine, which can cause a rash or act as a photosensitizer.

Tannic acid soothes severe sunburn. Apply used tea bags to the skin or remove the dark brown inner bark from an oak, chestnut, or hemlock tree and boil to make a tannic acid solution. Oatmeal, talcum powder, cornstarch, baking soda, and calamine are also soothing, especially if made into a cool paste with a water base. And you can cut the stalks and stems of aloe plants and rub them on the sunburn.

If you have skin type I or II, or you spend a lot of time outdoors, have your doctor check you for skin cancer at least once a year. He can show you how to check yourself at monthly intervals. Remember, it's your hide!

〰 HEAT ILLNESS

It was unusually warm for the opening day of deer season, warmer than Jim had expected it to be. By noon he had brought down a nice nine-point buck, dressed it out, and started out on the three-mile trek back to camp. After a mile, the sweat was pouring out of him like water out of a fountain. He stopped to rest under the sparse shade of a white oak, and peeled off his sweat-drenched flannel shirt. He craved a drink of cold water, but all he had was a thermos of coffee. He emptied it to lighten his load a bit, shouldered the deer, and continued on his way.

The cramps started as hard knots in his calves. At first he tried to ignore them. But after struggling over a high ridge with the 180-pound deer on his back, he started to get terrific charleyhorses in his thighs. It felt as though his legs were going to explode. And now he was sweating buckets. He stopped at the top of the ridge to catch his breath and massage his legs.

Jim couldn't understand it. He'd hauled bigger deer out of these woods without working up a sweat. And at thirty, he was strong as a horse and considered himself to be in good physical shape.

As his heavy breathing subsided, he heard the soft babbling of a mountain brook. He got up and followed the sound down into a ravine a few yards away. He hobbled down the slope and dropped to his knees at the edge of a narrow stream. He thrust his head into the crystalline spring water, gulping down huge mouthfuls of the sweet liquid. When he had slaked his thirst, he filled the thermos and returned to the ridge-top. He broke open a bag of potato chips and hungrily devoured them. Then he laid back against a log and rested.

When he got back up on his feet a half-hour later, he was surprised to find that the cramps had disappeared. He loaded the deer onto his shoulders and was back in camp an hour later.

Jim had a classic case of *heat cramps*. Heat cramps are the least serious of a group of conditions known as *heat-related illnesses*.

Handling the Heat

The body combats heat stress in two ways. Sweating is the first line of defense. The human body can withstand extreme heat and humidity as long as the sweating mechanism is intact and the salt and water lost in sweat are replenished. Heat is lost as sweat evaporates from the skin surface. As the body adapts, or acclimatizes, to heat and humidity, it develops the ability to produce sweat with a lower concentration of sodium chloride. And the acclimatized individual can produce a greater quantity of sweat. Acclimatization generally takes 4 to 7 days.

The body's other major defense mechanism against heat stress is the dilation of blood vessels in the skin. This allows for greater dissipation of heat through convection, radiation, and conduction.

?❧ HEAT CRAMPS

Like most people who develop heat cramps, Jim was in good physical condition. However, he was not acclimatized to the hot weather he experienced on the first day of deer season. His body couldn't handle the extra heat his muscles generated by hauling a large deer across rough terrain on an unseasonably warm day. As a result, he sweated profusely and lost a large amount of salt (sodium chloride) in his sweat. The decreased sodium concentration in his blood caused his muscles to become more contractile, to the point where they went into spasm, which Jim felt as cramps. But he had the sense to rest, and was lucky enough to find the mountain stream. The potato chips he ate were loaded with salt, thus completing the restoration of the salt and water he had lost in his sweat.

Unlike victims of heatstroke, those who develop heat cramps sweat normally, and their body temperature doesn't rise. Heat cramps generally occur only in individuals who are in good physical condition.

?? HEAT EDEMA

Hormonal fluctuations and dilation of the blood vessels in the extremities and skin cause an expansion of the blood volume, which leads to edema (swelling) of the hands, feet, ankles, and legs. This is typically seen in unacclimated persons and the elderly. No treatment is needed, as the edema goes away in a few days.

?? HEAT SYNCOPE

In military circles, this is known as "the parade ground faint." The classic case is the recruit who faints after standing at attention for a prolonged period on a hot, humid day. This can happen to a fly fisherman or any unacclimated person under the right environmental conditions. There are several causes:

1. Loss of blood volume due to excess sweating.
2. Pooling of blood in the extremities after long periods of standing or sitting.
3. Dilation of the blood vessels in the skin and extremities.

The heat syncope victim doesn't really need any treatment. He usually comes to after lying on the ground for a few moments. You can avoid heat syncope by avoiding prolonged sitting or standing in hot weather.

?? HEAT EXHAUSTION

Heat exhaustion (heat prostration, heat collapse) is the most common form of heat illness. It afflicts unacclimatized people, whether physically active or sedentary, during periods of high temperature and humidity (temperatures over 90 degrees F, relative humidity over 60 percent). Older people on diuretics are especially prone to develop this syndrome, as are obese people.

If Jim had been in his fifties or sixties, and had been hunting on a hot, sticky day, he might have experienced sudden weakness, dizziness, headache, nausea, vomiting, sweating, and the urge to defecate in addition to his muscle cramps. He would collapse, and his skin would be cold and clammy and look ashen-gray. However, his temperature would remain normal or even slightly below normal. If he were taken to a cool spot and placed in a recumbent position, he could be expected to recover within an hour or two. The cool spring water would hasten his recuperation, but he'd revive without it.

The problem in victims of heat exhaustion isn't so much the loss of salt and water as it is a failure of the heart and blood vessels to respond appropriately to the heat. Although loss of salt and water in the sweat is not the primary problem in individuals with heat exhaustion, the syndrome can be prevented by drinking plenty of water and cola drinks, which contain high concentrations of sodium. In any event, recovery should be spontaneous if the victim is brought to a cool spot and placed in a recumbent position.

?? EXERTIONAL HEAT INJURY

No one who watched the finish of the women's marathon in the 1984 Los Angeles Olympics will soon forget the Swiss runner who wobbled and lurched like a rubber woman down the home stretch and barely made it across the finish line before collapsing. After running over twenty-six miles on a hot, humid day, she had developed *exertional heat injury*. This relatively uncommon condition is seen only in individuals who exercise strenuously on hot, humid days. Unlike classic heatstroke, the victims of exertional heat injury sweat freely. Unlike victims of heat cramps and heat exhaustion, these people have elevated body temperatures, usually in the 102 to 104 degree F range. In addition, they are likely to develop headache, gooseflesh on the chest and arms, chills, hyperventilation, nausea, vomiting, muscle cramps, loss of coordination, unsteady gait, and incoherent speech. They may pass out. In severe conditions, there may be damage to blood cells, muscles, blood vessels, and the kidneys.

The treatment of exertional heat injury, which must be instituted promptly to avoid these complications, consists of placing the victim under cold, wet sheets, massaging the arms and legs to improve the circulation, and giving fluids by mouth. He should be evacuated to a hospital as quickly as possible.

?◆ HEATSTROKE

Heatstroke (sunstroke) is rarely suffered by young people. It primarily afflicts older people with chronic medical problems, especially heart disease, diabetes, and alcoholism. Contrary to popular belief, direct exposure to the sun is not necessary to develop heatstroke.

In heatstroke, the victim loses the ability both to sweat and to dilate the blood vessels under the skin. As a result, he has no effective means to dissipate body heat, and may suddenly collapse. Alternatively, he may complain of headache, dizziness, faintness, confusion, rapid breathing, and sometimes delirium before becoming lethargic and then comatose. The typical victim of heatstroke is confused or unconscious, and has an elevated body temperature (usually over 106 degrees F) and warm, dry skin.

Once body temperature exceeds 106 degrees, the blood and internal organs, especially the brain, heart, kidneys, and liver, start to bake. Only heroic methods can prevent death. The heatstroke victim needs to be cooled rapidly. Remove most of his clothing and place him in an ice-water bath, if possible, or some other cool place, such as a lake or stream. If a bath or body of water isn't available, apply ice packs to his neck, groin, armpits and chest, and cover him with cold wet towels under a fan. After his temperature has been lowered to 102 degrees, place him in a cool, well-ventilated place and massage his skin. This stimulates the flow of cool blood from the skin to the overheated internal organs, and the return of warm blood from these organs to the skin, where its heat is dissipated. As soon as he is alert, give the victim cold fluids by mouth. And arrange for speedy medical evacuation.

97

❧ PREVENTION OF HEAT ILLNESS

Here's how to stay cool when the going gets hot:

1. Take a few days to become acclimatized to a hot climate before embarking on an arduous hike or climb.
2. Stay hydrated. You can easily lose a liter or two of sweat an hour while exercising in a hot, humid environment. And you will lose even more after you acclimate. To prevent dehydration, you should drink 500 ml of water before and 200 to 300 ml every 15 to 20 minutes during exercise. The sodium, chloride, and potassium lost in sweat are generally adequately replaced with meals or snacks. (Forget about salt tablets. They irritate the stomach and cause vomiting.) Gatorade and similar commercial solutions are excellent rehydrating solutions. You can make your own weak electrolyte solution by adding 3–4 tsp of sugar and ½ tsp of salt to a liter of water. Drink it cold and it will be absorbed quicker.
3. Wear light-colored, loose-fitting clothing. Light colors absorb less light, and flowing clothing allows maximal evaporative heat loss. Did you ever see a Bedouin wearing tight-fitting, black clothing?
4. Take frequent dips in cold-water streams or lakes.
5. Accelerate evaporative heat loss after exercising in hot weather by dipping your clothes in water.
6. Remain in a cool environment as much as possible, and avoid the midday sun.

11

LIGHTNING INJURIES

"It is the mountaintop that the lightning strikes."

HORACE, *Odes*

❧

Does lightning strike twice? You bet. Shenandoah Park Ranger Roy Sullivan was zapped seven times in thirty-five years. He survived all seven strikes, but lightning blew off one toenail, vaporized his eyebrows, ignited his hair (twice), and once blew him out of a moving car. No one knows just why Roy was a human lightning rod, but being an outdoorsman had something to do with it. Most lightning strikes occur in rural areas, and hikers, campers, and outdoor sportsmen are on the receiving end of most lightning injuries.

Hurricanes and earthquakes hog the headlines, but year in and year out, lightning accounts for more weather-related deaths than any other natural disaster. Lightning strikes hundreds of people in the United States each year, killing as many as 300. When you consider that there are 50,000 thunderstorms and 8 million lightning strikes (100 each second) each day around the world, it's a wonder that more of us aren't struck by lightning.

Lightning is an awesome force, capable of generating up to 300,000 amps of current and 2 billion volts of electrical potential. That's enough power to shift a five-ton boulder or blast a Douglas fir into toothpicks. You can imagine what it can do to a human being.

❧ LIGHTNING MYTHS AND SUPERSTITIONS

1. "The safest place to wait out a lightning storm outdoors is under a tree." Only if you're in the mood

for a little cosmic electroshock therapy. Lightning tends to strike the highest object in an area. If the tree you're standing under is hit by lightning, you're going to get zapped too.

2. "You'll always be safe from lightning in a car." Only if it's a hardtop. All-metal cars deflect the charge around the metal skin and down into the ground. Open-frame vehicles and convertibles won't protect you from lightning.

3. "Lightning never strikes on a clear day." Lightning can strike during a snowstorm, sandstorm, a volcanic eruption, or seemingly "out of the blue" when a long horizontal flash turns earthward miles from the cloud that spawned it.

4. "Lightning strike is usually fatal." Wrong. Lightning kills only about 30 percent of its victims, and timely CPR would save most of them.

5. "If you hear thunder, you're safe from lightning strike." Well, for a while, anyway, since lightning precedes thunder by several seconds. But you won't hear the one that hits you.

6. "It's dangerous to touch a lightning strike victim." Yes, if the victim is a rattlesnake. Otherwise, there is no problem. The electric current passes through the victim's body in a fraction of a second and is gone.

7. "Lightning injuries are no different from other electrical injuries." Lightning usually passes outside the body, so injuries are usually less severe than those caused by generated electricity, which traverses the body and damages internal organs.

8. "Lightning victims are in a state of 'suspended animation' and may be revived after prolonged resuscitation." You're thinking of cold-water immersion. Lightning confers no protective effect on brain metabolism. Breathing and heartbeat have to be restored within minutes to allow any chance for survival in a person who has been "struck dead."

9. "Lightning never strikes twice." If you don't believe the story about the park ranger, ask the guy who owns the Empire State building. It's hit by lightning thousands of times a year. And so are many mountain peaks and radio and television antennas. Whatever it is that attracts lightning to an object will attract it repeatedly.

๏ A STORM IS BORN

A thundercloud is a giant electrical generator, cranking out thousands of megawatts of juice with each lightning bolt. It all starts when a cold front (high-pressure system) collides with a warm front (low-pressure system). The warm, moist air rises over the cold air, forming a cumulonimbus (thunder) cloud as the moisture in the warm air condenses into water particles in the form of raindrops, snow, hail, and ice crystals. These particles collide and pick up electrical charges as they are whipped around by violent updrafts and downdrafts in the cloud. The negatively charged particles collect in the bottom of the cloud and the positively charged particles in the top of the cloud, creating an enormous electrical potential between the two regions. Air is a very poor conductor of electricity, so this potential can reach hundreds of millions of volts before the electrical energy is dissipated as lightning strikes within the cloud (*sheet lightning*) or from cloud to ground (*streak lightning*).

As the thundercloud scuds across the surface of the earth, the strong negative charge in the bottom of the cloud induces a positive charge in the normally negatively charged earth. When the electrical potential becomes great enough to overcome the insulating properties of the air between ground and cloud, there is a flash of lightning. (The positive charge created by the thundercloud can also make your hair crackle and stand on end, and is the force behind St. Elmo's Fire, the eerie, dancing blue or green lights seen in a boat's rigging or on an airplane's wing before a storm.)

Contrary to what your eyeballs tell you, lightning doesn't move just from cloud toward earth, but mostly from earth upward. That giant, forked spark that you see is called the *leader stroke* or "stepped ladder." It's a 30-million volt, 250,000-amp trailblazing stroke that moves relatively slowly toward the earth, creating a low-resistance pathway through the air. As it nears the ground, a *pilot stroke* rises to meet it. Then a powerful *return stroke* rockets up this low-resistance channel at half the speed of light. The flickering light you see during a thunderstorm is a rapid sequence of secondary leader and return strokes flashing between earth and cloud.

Lightning Morphology

Lightning can take odd forms. *Ribbon lightning* is streak lightning blown by the wind. *Pearl lightning* is a flash broken into segments. *Ball lightning* is an eerie luminescent ball, one to several inches in diameter, that can be downright weird. (In 1685, a "ball of fire" floated into a gun room aboard the Royal Navy ship *Coronation*. It knocked a boy overboard, rendered several men unconscious, scorched the ship's timbers, and broke several windows before dispersing itself on the deck.)

Thunder

Lightning is hot stuff. Hot enough to heat the air it passes through to about 50,000 degrees Fahrenheit (five times hotter than the surface of the sun) in a fraction of a second. The clap and rumble of thunder is *not* the sound of Henry Hudson's crew playing tenpins (as they like to say in the Hudson Valley), but is attributed to shock waves created by the explosively expanding air. (You can estimate the distance in miles to the flash by counting the number of seconds between lightning and thunder and dividing by five.)

?❧ LIGHTNING INJURIES

Mechanisms of Injury

Lightning can hit you in any of several ways. If you are caught out in the open during a lightning storm, you may be the victim of a *direct strike*. Wearing or carrying a metal object above shoulder level, such as a backpack, ice axe or rifle, makes you an inviting target for a lightning strike. A *contact injury* occurs when you're holding a tent pole or some other object that is struck by lightning. A *splash injury* (also called *side flash* or *spray current*) classically occurs when lightning, seeking the path of least resistance, jumps from a tree to a person seeking refuge near the tree. Or it may jump from person to person in a group. Lightning striking the earth or a body of water causes an electric current to spread outward from the point of impact in concentric waves. This *ground current* (*step voltage, stride voltage*) can strike groups of hikers or swimmers. And you can be seriously injured by the *blast effect* of exploding/imploding air as lightning passes through it.

The "Flashover Effect"

A typical lightning bolt packs more punch than a cruise missile: 30 million volts and 250,000 amps of electrical energy. You'd think anyone struck by lightning would be turned into charcoal. But they aren't, thanks to the "flashover effect." Lightning contact with the body is so brief (a millisecond or less) that there is usually not enough time for it to burn an entrance hole in the skin and pass internally. Instead, the current flashes over the outside of the body, vaporizing sweat and blasting off clothing and shoes. (Household current, on the other hand, causes the victim to "freeze" to the circuit. The skin is broken down and electricity surges through the tissues, baking internal organs.)

ᔯ SPECIFIC INJURIES

A lightning strike may blow your socks off, yet cause amazingly minor injuries, such as transient blindness and deafness, confusion, muscle pain, and concussion. A heavier jolt might knock you out, crack a few bones, and paralyze your limbs. Or it might "strike you dead."

Cardiopulmonary

Lightning acts like a massive cosmic countershock, triggering a prolonged contraction of the heart muscle, followed by cardiac standstill for a brief period. It also paralyzes the breathing center in the brain. Death is not instantaneous, though. The heart almost always resumes beating soon after the shock. But the brain takes longer to recover; after going without oxygen for a few minutes, the heart goes into ventricular fibrillation, and the victim dies of this "secondary cardiac arrest" unless a rescuer gives him mouth-to-mouth ventilation.

Central Nervous System

A lightning strike to the head is like a Mike Tyson punch. With brass knuckles. It can fracture your skull and scramble your brains, leaving you confused and amnesic for days. It can cause subdural and epidural hematomas (intracranial bleeding). It may knock you out, leave you stunned, confused, and amnesic, and it may even change your personality. Two out of three lightning victims have transient paralysis of the legs, and one third will have paralyzed arms. Not surprisingly, lightning victims often develop a phobia of storms.

Burns

Flashover protects the skin from deep burns, but you may be scorched by belt buckles, jewelry, coins, or keys superheated by the lightning. Or the lightning may leave its calling card in the form of *feathering burns,* leaflike patterns where the skin has been imprinted by electron showers.

Circulation

Spasm of the blood vessels can cause the limbs to turn blue, mottled, and cold. Pulses in the arms and legs may be diminished.

Ears

The intense noise of thunder, which at ground zero approximates the sound of a battleship falling off a fifty-story building, can cause temporary deafness. The shock wave or skull fracture may rupture your eardrums and cause vertigo and impaired balance.

Eyes

Lightning can cause a wide range of eye injuries, including transient or permanent blindness, corneal injuries, retinal detachment, bleeding into the front or back chamber of the eye, double vision, degeneration of the optic nerves, and loss of color vision. Cataracts are common, and usually develop within a few days of injury. Lightning also can cause the pupils to become widely dilated and unresponsive to light. Fixed, dilated pupils are not a sign of death in a lightning victim.

Blast Effect

The explosive force of lightning may rupture the liver, spleen or kidneys, or blow you off a horse or a mountain ledge, causing you to fracture your ribs, skull, limbs, spine, or pelvis.

?? TREATMENT

Recognizing Lightning Injury

Lightning strikes in the flash of an eye, and if you aren't on the scene when it happens, you may be unsure of whether you are dealing with the victim of a seizure, stroke, heart attack, drug overdose, or foul play. If you come across a person lying unconscious in an open field with his clothes in shreds and bruises all over his body, you might logically conclude that he's been assaulted. But if he is unconscious or dazed, has burns in a feather or leaflike pattern on his skin, has blood draining from his ears, and his arms and legs are cold, blue and mottled, you can safely assume that he's been struck by lightning.

First Response

The Home Cookbook in 1877 gave its readers this advice:

> "TO RESTORE FROM STROKE OF LIGHTNING. Shower with cold water for two hours; if the patient does not show signs of life, put salt in the water, and shower an hour longer."

Why don't you just skip that and remember the ABCs: airway, breathing, and circulation. If the victim isn't breathing and has no pulse, start CPR. If you are successful in restoring a heartbeat, continue breathing for the victim until he starts breathing on his own. (This might be several minutes or longer.) Then do a systematic search for other injuries, making sure that you keep his neck and back immobilized if you have reason to suspect spinal injury. Splint any fractures, attend to any wounds or burns, and treat for hypothermia if he's been exposed to the elements for any length of time.

Group Therapy

Mass casualties are traditionally "triaged"—that is, sorted into three groups:

1. Those victims who are going to survive no matter what is done for them.
2. Those who are going to die no matter what is done for them.
3. Those who are going to die if something isn't done for them *right now*.

Then, the first two groups are ignored until those in the last group are stabilized. But the rules change when you're dealing with a group of people who have been struck by lightning. Now, you *"resuscitate the dead."* People who are moaning and groaning are going to make it. Those in cardiac arrest have a good chance for survival if they are given CPR, particularly if you get to them before the heart goes into "secondary arrest" due to lack of oxygen. (Remember, if you are able to restore a heartbeat, prolonged artificial breathing may be necessary.) Then, go back to the ABCs as you evaluate and treat the other victims and prepare them for evacuation. Wounds, fractures and dislocations, burns, head injuries, chest and abdominal injuries are treated in the usual way. Ruptured eardrums don't require immediate treatment, but do require eventual medical evaluation. Many eye injuries will also (see Chapter 7). Cold, blue extremities are often a sign of shock or hypothermia, but in this setting are probably due to vascular spasm, and should regain their normal color and temperature within a few hours. Naturally, if there are other signs of shock, treat them as such. Paralysis after lightning strikes normally resolves also within a few hours. If it doesn't, you'll have to assume that the victim has a brain or spinal cord injury and arrange for medical evacuation.

ঌ OUT OF HARM'S WAY: AVOIDING LIGHTNING INJURY

Lightning is one of nature's great spectacles, but you don't want to become part of the show. Here's how to stay out of trouble during a thunderstorm:

- Seek refuge in a building or an all-metal vehicle.
- If you see St. Elmo's fire on nearby objects (or yourself), or feel your hair standing on end, hit the deck.
- Stay out of tents (tent poles can be lightning rods).
- Put down guns or other metal objects, remove metal objects from your hair, take off hobnailed boots, and stay away from fences, power lines, and pipelines.
- If you are in a forest, wait out the storm in a low area under a thick growth of small trees.
- If you are in the open, stay away from single trees, corn stalks, and hay stacks. Find a dry cave or a ditch, and crouch down with your feet close together. Or lie curled up on the ground on a rubber or plastic raincoat.
- If you are with a group of people, spread out to avoid ground current and splashes.

If you are on the water in a small boat, the sound of thunder rolling across the bay may be the Heavenly Trumpeter calling you home to your Maker if you don't act quickly. Your first move should be toward the ignition or the oars. Get under way and head for shore.

If you are offshore, look for a sailboat or a large cabin cruiser. You can pull alongside and ride out the storm under its cone of protection. If you are near shore, you can take refuge under a bridge or cliff. But stay inside the cabin if you have one, or hunker down in the bottom of the boat. Keep your hands off the railings, windshield frame, radio antennas, stern light, fishing reels, outriggers, and downriggers. Anything metallic will attract lightning, so remove your jewelry and belt buckles and empty the change from your pockets. Pump the bilge, and keep your feet out of the water. Lightning will take the path of least resistance through a boat, and has been known to travel through water-filled hoses leading from the head to through-hull fittings and blow people off toilet seats. Stay out of the head. And stay out of the water. Groups of people in the water have been killed by ground current.

A sailboard is a lightning rod on a surfboard. If you can't get to shore quickly, just let the mast and sail go over and lie down on the board.

Aluminum is an excellent conductor of electricity, and an aluminum boat is a magnet for lightning. Sitting out a thunderstorm in an aluminum boat is like waiting out a forest fire in an ammunition dump. Not only are you vulnerable to a direct strike, but lightning striking the water anywhere within 100 yards can spread to your boat in the form of lethal ground current.

Fiberglass, on the other hand, is such a poor conductor of electricity that it acts as an electrical insulator. But that doesn't make your fiberglass boat lightning-proof. That same quality can transform it into a giant capacitor. A capacitor, you may remember, is a device that stores electricity. It consists of a nonconductor separating conductors carrying opposite electrical charges. A thundercloud passing overhead induces a positive charge in the people in the boat. This positive charge builds up until the electrical potential between people and water (ground, negatively charged) overcomes the resistance of the fiberglass, and a powerful current flows through the hull into the water, injuring or killing those on board.

Graphite and boron are electrical conductors, so fishing rods made of these materials can act as hand-held lightning rods. And so can a wet fiberglass rod. Most fishing lines are nonconductors, but water is a good conductor of electricity. Lightning hitting the water can flash up a wet line and shock the fisherman holding the rod. Reel in your line and get those sticks down the minute you see a thunderstorm approaching.

12

DROWNING AND NEAR-DROWNING

*"Lord, Lord! methought, what pain it was to drown:
What dreadful noise of waters in my ears!
What ugly sights of death within my eyes!
Methought I saw a thousand fearful wracks;
A thousand men that fishes gnaw upon."*

—SHAKESPEARE,
Richard III

Take it from me, drowning is a very unpleasant business. I fell into a well when I was a little shaver, and I'll never forget the few moments I spent in that murky water, thrashing about wildly, desperately grabbing for something to hang onto, sucking huge mouthfuls of water into my lungs before I blacked out. My dad happened to come along, spotted my cowboy hat floating on the surface of the water, and pulled me out by the hair just as I was sinking out of reach. It was an experience I hope never to repeat.

About 9,000 people die by drowning in the United States every year. Another 80,000 have near-misses, like mine. Drowning is the second-leading cause of accidental death in those under age 45. You can drown in a well, and you can drown in a puddle. A guy in Australia drowned in a wash bucket. And being a good swimmer won't always save you from a watery grave.

Let's define a few terms before we get in over our heads. *Immersion* is the state of being in the water with your head out. *Submersion* is the state of being under the water, head and all. *Aspiration* is the inhalation of water or stomach contents into the lungs. *Drowning* is death by asphyxia following submersion. *Near-drowning* is at least temporary survival after being submersed.

Predisposing Factors

Inability to swim is an obvious risk factor for drowning. Here are a few more:

1. *Head and neck injury.* It is impossible to swim with a broken neck and paralyzed limbs. Head-first dives into shallow water and underwater obstructions are the number-one cause of cervical spinal cord injuries. Look before you leap!

2. *Alcohol and other drugs.* An Australian study showed that 64 percent of men who drowned had been drinking prior to the event. As little as two beers can slow reaction time, dull your reflexes, and impair your judgment. Three or four beers will give you blurred or tunnel vision, decrease your coordination, and make you more susceptible to exhaustion, hypothermia, and cardiac arrest in cold water. So-called recreational drugs cloud your sensorium and impair your decision-making ability.

3. *Hypothermia.* You can become hypothermic in any water that's cooler than 77 degrees if you're in it long enough. Hypothermia saps your strength and stiffens your muscles. How are you going to climb back into a boat or up a muddy embankment if your muscles feel like Play Doh?

4. *Seizures.* If you're epileptic, you know that a seizure can strike at any time. You'll be between the devil and the deep blue sea if you have one while in the water.

5. *Hyperventilation.* Remember how, when you were a kid, you used to try to knock your pal out by getting him to hyperventilate? If you hyperventilate before swimming underwater, you can develop "shallow-water blackout." Rapid breathing lowers the carbon dioxide content of the blood, removing the stimulus to breathe. As you continue to swim underwater, you use up oxygen. When the blood oxygen content gets low enough, the light bulb goes out and you drown.

6. *Gender.* Males dominate the drowning statistics. In boating-related drownings, male victims outnumber females 12 to 1.

The Physiology of Drowning

The process of drowning is an action-packed series of events. Here's what happens:

1. First you panic. You kick, scream, and thrash about like a wild man. (The first thing they taught me when I became a lifeguard was how to approach

and subdue a drowning person. We mastered the half-Nelson before we swam a stroke.)

2. All that to-do makes you too tired to keep your head above water, so you start holding your breath. (You also swallow lots of water, which distends your stomach and makes you vomit.)

3. When you can hold your breath no longer, you start gasping for air, and inhale enough water to block your airway. This leads to a severe drop in blood oxygen content, and you pass out, aspirate more water, and suffocate if you're not pulled from the water and resuscitated in time. When the brain goes without oxygen for more than 4 or 5 minutes, it's damaged irreversibly, and when the heart is deprived of oxygen for that length of time, it fibrillates. (Curiously, about 15 percent of drowning victims have such intense spasm of the vocal cords that they don't aspirate *any* water. This is called "dry drowning." In the other 85 percent of drowning cases, the lungs are filled with water. This is called "wet drowning.")

Fresh Water Aspiration

Fresh water is *hypotonic* relative to plasma, the liquid component of blood. That means that it has a lower concentration of salts dissolved in it. When a few mouthfuls of fresh water are aspirated, osmosis pulls some of it across the inner surface of the lungs into the bloodstream, and then into the red blood cells. This dilutes the blood, and may stretch the red blood cells until they pop (this is called "hemolysis").

Fresh water also inactivates "surfactant" and washes it out of the lungs. Surfactant is a surface-tension-lowering substance that coats the inner surface of the lung and prevents the small air cells in the lung from collapsing, in much the same way that soap added to water decreases its surface tension and allows you to blow bubbles. As these air cells collapse, the oxygen content of the blood decreases and the lungs become stiff, increasing the work of breathing.

Seawater Aspiration

Seawater is salty, of course. So is the blood, but seawater contains a much greater concentration of sodium, chloride, and other salts than does plasma, and so is *hypertonic* relative to plasma. Rather than being drawn into the bloodstream, aspirated seawater draws plasma into the lungs, causing the air cells to become fully saturated with water. The flow of plasma out of the bloodstream and into the lungs causes a drop in blood pressure and concentration of the blood.

Seawater doesn't inactivate surfactant, but it does wash it out of the air cells.

Brackish Water

Brackish water may contain any number of pollutants that can sear the lungs and cause an intense inflammatory pneumonia. It's also more likely to contain sand, seaweed, mud, and sewage. This material can be aspirated and obstruct the airway.

Freshwater and seawater cause different insults, but practically speaking, it doesn't make a drop of difference whether the submersion incident occurs in salt, fresh, or brackish water. The near-drowning victim is treated precisely the same, whether he was pulled out of the surf at Montauk or fished out of the Snake River in Idaho.

The Immersion Syndrome

Jumping into icy water can cause instant death, right? Well, sometimes. The shock of cold water on the skin causes a reflex gasp, which can cause you to inhale a lungful of water and drown. Or it may cause a reflex slowing of the heartbeat that leads to cardiac arrest. But most people survive for up to an hour even in 0 degree C (32 degrees F) water.

Cold-Water Drowning

There have been recent reports of children who were successfully resuscitated after being submerged in cold water for as long as 66 minutes. It was once thought that victims of cold-water submersion are protected by a primitive "diving reflex" that slows the heartbeat, closes down the airway, and shunts blood to the brain. Seals have such a reflex, but there is no evidence that humans do. It's now believed that these cold-water submersion survivors underwent such severe and rapid cooling that they were in a "metabolic icebox" that protected the brain from permanent injury. Adults, having lower surface-to-mass ratios, cool too slowly to be protected this way.

Basic Lifesaving

The first rule for any would-be rescuer is to not become a victim yourself. Panic can endow the drowning person with the power of Samson. If you jump into the water and swim right out to him, he is liable to crawl right on top of you.

The safest approach to the person in distress in the water is to extend a long stick, rope, or pole out to him. Let him grab the end and pull himself in. If a rope is handy, throw it to him, and pull him in.

If the victim is too far out to reach with a stick or rope, and you are trained in water rescue techniques, you are going to have to swim out and get him. Here is a review of the basic techniques:

1. If the victim is rational and cooperative, you can use the *tired swimmer's carry*. Approach him from the front, and tell him to put his hands on your shoulders. Then use the breaststroke to return to shore.

2. If the victim is flailing wildly, swim to him underwater, turn him around so that he is facing away from you, and raise his head out of the water by lifting on his hips. Next, place your hand under his jaw to keep his head out of the water, and allow his body to level off. Then, reach your arm around his chest and sidestroke to shore. If he panics, join your hands and just keep his face out of the water until he calms down. Or escape by letting go of him and sinking down into the water.

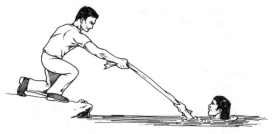

17. *Rescuing the near-drowning victim from the shore.*

18. *Rescuing the near-drowning victim with a branch or log.*

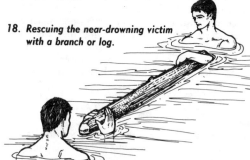

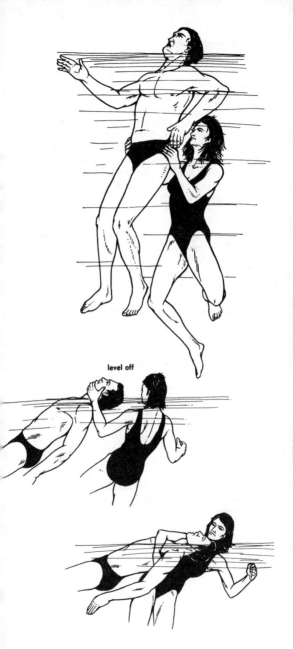

level off

19. The "cross-chest" carry.

Treatment

What would you do if you pulled a near-drowning victim from the water? Roll him over a barrel? Throw him onto a horse and trot him around? Those were state-of-the-art resuscitation techniques in the seventeenth and eighteenth centuries. Nowadays, drainage procedures are considered useless and dangerous. Attention is focused instead on the ABCs (*A*irway, *B*reathing, and *C*irculation), stabilizing and protecting the cervical spine, placing the victim on his side or in a prone position so that he doesn't aspirate his stomach contents, and rewarming him if he is hypothermic.

If the victim is in cardiac arrest, start CPR as soon as you get him on shore or into a boat (see Chapter 1). If the airway is blocked, perform the Heimlich maneuver or remove mud and debris manually. Continue CPR until you revive the victim or emergency medical personnel take over. If you're in the wilderness, continue CPR until the victim has warmed to ambient temperature. Remember, the cold-water drowning victim is not dead until he's warm and dead.

The Postimmersion Syndrome

Some near-drowning victims appear to be fine after they are pulled out of the water, but may develop severe shortness of breath minutes to hours after the incident. This is called "secondary drowning" or the "postimmersion syndrome." It probably represents the delayed effect of inactivation or washout of surfactant from the lungs, damage to the air cells, or an inflammatory response to chemicals in the water. Anyone who has been submersed for more than a minute or two should be evaluated medically and observed for onset of the postimmersion.

If you spend a lot of time on the water, you should consider taking a Red Cross lifesaving course. Armed with that, a CPR course, and a little common sense, you should do swimmingly.

13

INSECT, SPIDER, AND SCORPION BITES AND STINGS

"When I get sick of what men do, I have only to walk a few steps in another direction to see what spiders do."

—ELWYN BROOKS WHITE

"This is the Black Widow, death."

—ROBERT LOWELL, *Mr. Edwards and the Spider*

❧ SPIDERS

I don't know about you, but I don't like spiders. Maybe it was the science fiction movie I saw as a kid. The one where giant spiders, ugly things with eight eyes and fur all over their bodies, terrorize a small town, eating the sheriff and a couple of his deputies before moving on to the grade school to scarf down a bunch of little kids.

Or maybe it was all those stories about the wicked black widow that prejudiced me against her kind. How one bite can kill you, and how she eats her spouse after mating. And the stories we used to hear about tarantulas made the black widow look like a harmless spinster.

No matter what your feelings about these creatures, you should know that there are about 50 species of poisonous spiders in the United States. The two most dangerous spiders found in the United States, the black widow and the brown recluse, hang out under stones, logs and bark, in clumps of vegetation, in fields, vineyards, woods, and in barns, sheds, outhouses, and other buildings. Everywhere a hunter might go.

Spiders are arachnids, a class that includes scorpions, ticks, and centipedes. They live everywhere and are prodigious travelers, the hobos of the arachnid world. Up to 2 million may live in an acre of grassland, 265,000 in an acre of woodland.

Spiders have two major body segments, the cephalothorax and the abdomen, eight legs, a pair of feelers, and a pair of jaws. At the end of each jaw is a hollow fang, which connects to a venom sac in the cephalothorax. Spider venom contains potent chemicals which paralyze and partially digest prey.

Spiders are meat eaters, dining mostly on other insects. The larger ones also feast on frogs, lizards, and fish. Most spiders are harmless to humans, but about a dozen of the thousands of species that make their home in the United States can cause at least mild illness. The bites of some can be fatal.

℘ THE BLACK WIDOW SPIDER

Latrodectus mactans, the infamous black widow, is found throughout the United States and southern Canada. The dangerous female is the size (excluding the legs) of a thumbnail and has a shiny, coal black body, a prominent, spherical stomach, and a characteristic red or orange hourglass marking on her undersurface. The male is half the size of the female, too small to have a harmful bite.

Like venomous snakes, the black widow is not aggressive toward humans, and attacks only when she or her web is threatened. Her venom is more potent than that of a cobra or coral snake but, happily, she doesn't inject that much of it into her human victims.

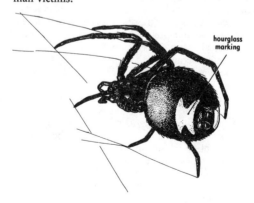

hourglass
marking

20. *The black widow spider, showing the characteristic hourglass marking.*

After mating with and then eating her husband (when she can catch him), the female finds a dark corner, weaves a coarse web, and suspends her eggs in it. Although generally regarded as timid, black widows defend their eggs the way a grizzly mother defends her cubs. She can be downright nasty. In the days before indoor plumbing, half the reports of black widow spider bites involved men bitten on the genitals while sitting in outhouses.

Bite Signs and Symptoms

For all its fearsome reputation, the black widow spider bite is initially painless and invisible; you may not even realize that you've been bitten. Fifteen minutes later, you'll start to feel as jumpy as a cat on a hot tin roof. Painful cramps in the area around the bite will spread up your arm or leg and then throughout your body. Sweat will pour out of you, and your temperature and blood pressure will head north. You'll look like you're in shock, with a weak, thready pulse, cold, clammy skin, shortness of breath, and slurred speech. If you're bitten in the leg or genitals, your abdomen will become rigid as a board, and you may get taken off to the operating room for an operation you don't need. If you're bitten on the arm, you'll get terrific spasms of the chest muscles and pain that mimics a heart attack. And you may get a weird burning sensation on the soles of your feet, a splitting headache, dizziness, difficulty swallowing, nausea, vomiting, swelling of the face, and droopy eyelids that a bloodhound would envy.

That's the bad news. The good news is that black widow spider bites are rarely fatal. You may want to die at first, but after a few hours the cramps start to subside, and you'll be back to normal in two or three days.

Treatment

First aid for the black widow bite victim consists of cleansing the bite wound and application of cold packs. Then you'd better head for the nearest hospital, where they'll give you an injection of calcium gluconate or methocarbamol, a muscle relaxant. Antivenin is reserved for serious envenomations in children, the elderly, and pregnant women. Hot baths may help as well. Cutting and suctioning *never* work.

Avoid this wrathful woman by wearing long-sleeved shirts and pants when you are in country known to be inhabited by black widows, and watch where you sit!

૨ **BROWN SPIDERS**

Loxosceles spiders, the brown recluse and its cousins, are much more of a threat to outdoorsmen than black widows. There are more of them, both sexes bite, and their bites can cause "necrotic arachnidism": gangrenous ulcers, systemic poisoning, and even death.

Identification

The brown recluse is a deceptively innocent-appearing, medium-sized, fawn to dark-brown spider. It has a characteristic violin-shaped figure on its back, and is known as the "fiddle-back" spider. It ranges throughout the United States, but prefers hot, arid environments. True to its name, it remains secluded during the day, venturing out at night to hunt beetles, flies, and other spiders. During these nightly forays, it sometimes finds its way into bedding or clothing, thus setting the scene for a spider-man encounter of the worst kind!

Bite Signs and Symptoms

The bite of the brown spider may be virtually painless. More commonly, it causes a sharp, stinging pain that intensifies over a period of 6 to 8 hours, turning into a terrific ache as chemicals in the venom constrict the blood vessels in the area of the bite, shutting off blood flow to the skin and underlying fat. The skin around the bite swells and a large, violet

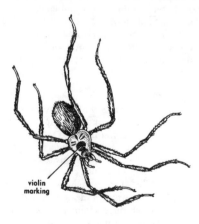

violin
marking

21. *The brown recluse spider, showing the characteristic violin marking.*

blister develops. This blister becomes progressively darker over the next 24 to 72 hours and turns into a thick black scab. The scab sloughs off after a few weeks, leaving a deep ulcer.

Severe bites can be associated with fever, joint pains, rash, weakness, nausea, and vomiting. Children may have an especially severe reaction in which red blood cells and blood platelets are destroyed, resulting in anemia and a bleeding tendency.

Treatment

Brown spider bites can't be effectively treated in the wild. The best thing to do is to apply cold packs to the bite, elevate and immobilize the bitten extremity, and head for a hospital.

Excision of the bite was once considered standard treatment for brown spider bites, but neither that nor cortisone injections have been shown to be of any value. The most promising approach appears to be a combination of antivenin (still experimental) injected directly into the bite, antibiotics, and dapsone, a drug used to treat leprosy. Dapsone inhibits the influx of white blood cells into the area of the bite, and this in some unknown way counteracts the effects of the venom. Skin grafting is often needed to repair the necrotic ulcer.

Prevention

Brown spiders can be controlled by cleaning up piles of wood and other debris and spraying sheds and outbuildings with a carbamate insecticide. The most practical advice for outdoorsmen is to shake out your bedding and clothing in the morning.

?❧ TARANTULAS

Bird spiders, funnel-web spiders, and trapdoor spiders are *tarantulas,* big, furry spiders that live long and move slowly. About forty species of tarantulas are native to the United States. Their bites resemble bee stings, and require nothing more than elevation, immobilization, and a couple of aspirins.

?❧ WOLF SPIDERS

Lycosidae are a family of hunting spiders that roam through fields and pastures looking for prey. Most wolf spiders found in the United States cause a mild, stinging bite that requires nothing more than local wound care, ice, and elevation.

୬ SCORPIONS

If any bug can rival the black widow's sinister reputation, it's the scorpion. This primitive arachnid stung more than 2,375 humans in 1985, sending 403 of them to the hospital. To put the problem in perspective, only 245 people were treated for snakebite that year. None of these bites were fatal, but 188 were described as moderate to severe.

Identification

Scorpions are easy to identify. They look like small lobsters, with an elongated abdominal segment that curves up over the body and ends in a *telson*, which contains a stinging apparatus.

Nocturnal animals, scorpions burrow in the sand or hide in fallen trees, under rocks and logs, in piles of wood or brush, or beneath houses and outbuildings during the day, and forage for insects, spiders, and other scorpions at night. Like their spider cousins, scorpions have poor vision. They rely instead on their sense of feel, stinging any moving object that touches or steps on them.

Scorpions hibernate in the winter, and are most active May through August.

Sting Signs and Symptoms

Nonlethal scorpions, such as *Vejovis spinigeris*, *Hadrurus arizonensis* and most *Centuroides* species, are denizens of the Great Sonoran Desert in Arizona and New Mexico and rarely cause more than a mild sting. You may think you've been stung by a bee or wasp, and there may be a little redness at the sting site. These stings need only a cold pack and antihistamines.

Centruroides Exilicauda

This is the only scorpion that causes severe toxicity in the United States. These guys are heavy hitters. They were responsible for 69 fatalities in Arizona between 1929 and 1954.

Called the "bark scorpion" because of its yellow to brown coloration, *Centruroides exilicauda* is about three inches long, has a knob at the base of its stinger, and may have dark stripes down its back. Home is the Sonoran desert, but its range is spreading into southern California, Texas, and northern Mexico.

Centruroides venom is neurotoxic: it causes prolonged hyperstimulation of the nervous system. Its sting can pack a wallop, but most serious envenomations occur in children, the elderly, and those with high blood pressure. Most adult envenomations aren't serious, causing only mild pain for a few hours. At first, you may feel nothing more than a pricking sensation; it leaves no bite mark (swelling or discoloration indicates that the sting was caused by a nonlethal species).

In more severe envenomations, pain intensifies over a period of a few minutes to an hour, and the area becomes exquisitely sensitive to the touch. Tapping the sting site sends pain and tingling sensations shooting up the arm or leg. The victim becomes jumpy and jittery; children may flail about grotesquely, as though they are in pain, but usually are not. (This hyperactivity has been described as "break-dancing in bed.") They may appear to be convulsing, but are alert and can talk.

Other signs of severe scorpion envenomation include high blood pressure, headache, salivation, abdominal cramps and vomiting, muscle twitching, roving eye movements, temporary blindness, rapid pulse, heavy perspiration, and goose bumps. Children sometimes develop wheezing and may have trouble breathing.

Treatment

Mild stings can be treated with ice packs and aspirin or acetaminophen. If the victim starts to develop significant pain, he has a serious envenomation and needs to be brought to a hospital. Cold packs will help control the pain en route, but he may need intravenous medications to counteract the nervous system stimulating effects of the venom. An antivenin made from goat serum is available in Arizona, but has not yet been approved by the FDA and is still considered experimental. Initial reports indicate that it is safe and effective.

Don't let scorpions get your goat. Outdoorsmen can avoid these nasty critters by

- Wearing shoes when walking outside at night
- Shaking out shoes and clothing before dressing each morning, and sleeping bags before turning in at night
- Keeping hands out of potential scorpion hideouts, especially woodpiles, under rocks, logs, and tree bark.

?❧ MOSQUITOES

In the tropics, mosquitoes are feared as the carriers of such serious diseases as dengue, malaria, and yellow fever. In the United States, mosquitoes are just plain nuisances. Nevertheless, these whining, swarming hellions on wings can make life miserable for outdoor enthusiasts, as can their coastal cousins, the gnats.

The problem starts when a female mosquito, attracted by carbon dioxide and human sweat, alights on your skin and takes a meal. She drills that syringe-like nose under the skin and injects saliva that contains a substance that thins the blood in the area of the bite, a few proteins that can trigger an allergic reaction, and possibly a few microorganisms to boot.

Bite Signs and Symptoms

A itchy wheal is the skin's first reaction to being drilled by Madame Mosquito. Within 12 to 24 hours, the area becomes red, swollen, and more itchy.

Treatment

An ice pack will minimize the swelling and itching in the first few minutes after a mosquito bite. Calamine or antihistamine lotion will decrease redness and itching. More intense reactions may require diphenhydramine, 25 or 50 mg by mouth every 6 hours.

Prevention

The first line of defense against mosquitoes is insect repellents. Make sure you take along a generous supply when you venture into the wild during the summer months. Mosquitoes are nocturnal feeders, so try to be indoors or inside a tent before dusk when in mosquito country. And pitch that tent high and dry, away from the low, wet areas where mosquitoes breed.

A mosquito can easily slip its proboscis through the mesh of light clothing, so wear loose clothing, and pad it with leaves, bark, or grass. To protect your head and neck, tie off the arms and neck of your undershirt and slip it over your head. Keep it off your scalp by padding your head with bark or leaves, and cut slits for your eyes.

A campfire may be your salvation when in mosquito country. The smoke will usually keep them away.

?❧ BLACKFLIES

Blackflies are winged demons that take over the woods in many sections of the northern United States during the summer months. They breed in mountain streams, brooks and rivers, but the adult fly prefers open, sunny areas.

Blackflies are diurnal bloodsuckers and are attracted by dark, moving objects. Most bites are on the upper body, and leave large, bleeding puncture wounds. The bite then becomes red, swollen and painful, and it may take weeks for the weeping, crusted sores to heal. Treatment consists of local wound care. Insect repellents and everyday clothing don't deter these hombres when they attack in droves.

?❧ STINGING INSECTS

The average bee weighs about as much as a candle flame, but packs the firepower of an F-14. Instead of bomb racks, they have venom sacs attached to their stingers. The sting of a bee, wasp, hornet, yellow jacket, or ant (all members of the order Hymenoptera) means instant pain. It may also mean instant death if you are one of the many people who are allergic to bees.

Honeybees are kamikazes. Their barbed stingers and venom sacs remain embedded in the skin after stinging, and when they fly away, they are disemboweled, and soon die.

Sting Signs and Symptoms

If you disturb a nest, you're liable to be swarmed. The first bee on the scene releases *pheromones,* chemical signals that trigger aggressive behavior in other bees. One sting will cause pain, swelling, and redness. Multiple bee stings can cause massive swelling, vomiting and diarrhea, shortness of breath, shock, and collapse. One hundred to 200 stings can be fatal.

Allergic reactions to bees range in severity from hives, swelling of the face, lips and throat, nausea and dizziness, to severe shortness of breath and wheezing, shock, and respiratory arrest. Most allergic reactions develop within a few minutes, although they may be delayed as long as six hours.

Treatment

An ice cube placed over the sting site and elevation of the limb will suffice for the 99 percent of people who are not allergic to bees. "Sting sticks" containing a local anesthetic and antihistamine lotions may relieve some of the discomfort. A couple of aspirin or acetaminophen tablets will also help.

If you *are* allergic to bees, you'll need a shot of adrenaline and an antihistamine if you develop any sign of a severe reaction (wheezing, swelling of the face and throat, collapse). Kits are available (Ana-Kit, EpiPen) that have preloaded syringes of adrenaline and diphenhydramine tablets for emergencies. If you have had a severe bee sting reaction in the past, apply a light tourniquet just above the sting if it's on an arm or leg.

Bee stingers continue to pulsate and squeeze venom into the tissues, so they should be removed quickly. If you try to pinch or squeeze the stinger out, you will just empty the venom sac. Instead, use a needle or knife point to gently ease it out. Or you can scrape it out with a credit card.

Prevention

- Don't leave food out in the open. Yellowjackets are attracted to meat, fruits, and fruit syrup. And keep an eye on open drinks: if you swallow a yellowjacket, it can sting you in the esophagus or in the nether regions of your gastrointestinal tract.
- Take great pains to avoid hymenopteran nests, or you will *be* in great pain. Honeybees favor rock crevices and hollow trees; you'll see wasp nests hanging from trees; yellowjackets nest underground in animal burrows and tree stumps; fire ants are found throughout the southern United States in mound nests in open, grassy areas.
- Stay out of the way of bees or other hymenopterans flying in a straight line. They may be making a "beeline" to their nest and may become aggressive if they think you are blocking their way.
- If you have an encounter with a bee, don't slap at it. That will just make him mad. Do the smart thing—run. Take refuge in a tent, building, vehicle, or in a dark, shady area.
- Be especially wary of bees on cloudy days. Like most of us, they are more irritable when the sky is gray and it's threatening to rain.
- Keep your shoes on when walking around in the woods.
- If you have a history of bee-sting allergy, take a bee-sting kit along with you into the wilderness and don't hesitate to use it.

?✒ CENTIPEDES

Centipedes are ubiquitous in the United States, but the giant desert centipede is the one you want to watch out for. This six-inch monster uses his curved, hollow fangs to cause an intensely painful bite with localized swelling and redness over the sting site and inflammation of regional lymph glands. If he hangs on long enough to squirt an extra dollop of venom under your skin, the swelling and tenderness may persist for three weeks, and the skin around the fang marks may slough off.

Treatment consists of thorough washing of the bite with soap and water and application of an ice pack. Avoid centipede bites by checking out your shoes, clothing, and sleeping bag before use when in centipede country. Keep your fingers out of crevices, and leave every stone unturned.

?✒ MILLIPEDES

Millipedes aren't endowed with fangs and venom. They fend off perceived attackers by showering them with a disagreeable chemical spray, after the fashion of skunks. If this stuff gets on your skin it can cause an irritating rash. If it gets in your eyes, it's worse than irritating. It'll make you shed buckets of tears, and your lids will clamp down like bear traps. It can cause swelling of the whites of the eyes, corneal ulcers, and even blindness. Skin contact should be treated like a superficial burn: wash the area with soap and water and apply triple antibiotic cream. Anyone sprayed in the eyes with this millipede mist needs to have his eyes washed out with copious amounts of sterile water and then to be evaluated by a physician.

?✒ A NOTE ON INSECT REPELLENTS

Deet is the most effective topical insect repellent now available. It is effective against mosquitoes, chiggers, biting flies, ticks, and fleas, but *not* against bees, wasps, and other hymenopterans. It can be applied directly to skin, clothing, tents, screens, and sleeping bags. Deet's one drawback is that it is absorbed through the skin and can cause hives, skin rashes, and central nervous system damage when used for prolonged periods or in excessive amounts. But the new long-acting 35 percent solution has a polymer that prevents evaporation as well as skin absorption.

Rutgers 612 and *dimethylphthalate* repel both mosquitoes and ticks, while *citronella* gives short-term protection against mosquitoes.

Permethrin is a pesticide that can be sprayed onto clothing to protect against mosquitoes and lice. The best mosquito and tick protection can be had by treating your clothing with permethrin and applying 35 percent Deet solution to exposed skin.

If you don't have any chemical repellents, mud will give you some protection.

SNAKE AND
REPTILE BITES

"And the Lord God said unto the serpent, Because thou hast done this, thou art cursed above all cattle, and above every beast of the field; upon thy belly shalt thou go, and dust shalt thou eat all the days of thy life."

—Genesis 3:14

𝄢

The snake struck with the speed and ferocity of a cruise missile. Fred screamed as the serpent buried its fangs in his thigh. A hit-and-run artist, it was nothing more than a blurred flash of copper slithering into the undergrowth by the time he realized what had happened. He lay on the ground in agony, clutching his throbbing leg, fighting back a wave of panic. He was alone in the Chattahoochee National Forest in Georgia, hours away from the nearest hospital. He rested his rifle against a tree and reached into his pack for a knife.

𝄢

Snakes have been getting man into trouble since the Garden of Eden. Snakes taste human flesh 45,000 times each year in the United States; 8,000 of the perpetrators are venomous snakes. About a dozen of these snakebites are delivered with extreme prejudice: their victims die. And you don't have to go to Georgia to get snakebit. The limbless wonders inhabit every state except Maine, Alaska, and Hawaii, and call a wide range of terrains home, from desert and swamps to mountains. Many can swim or climb trees.

The Cast of Characters

Two families of venomous snakes are indigenous to the United States, the Elapidae, which include the eastern and western coral snake, and the Crotalidae, or pit vipers, which include copperheads, cottonmouths (water moccasins), and rattlesnakes.

⅍ PIT VIPERS

Although the eastern coral snake is far deadlier, pit vipers have the country blanketed from coast to coast, and are responsible for most of the snakebites reported in this country.

Identifying Marks—Snake Anatomy 101

You've got to be able to "get a make" on the snake that bites you, since treatment depends on the perpetrator's species. Pit vipers have four distinguishing characteristics:

1. A heat sensing *pit* between the eye and nostril on each side of the head. These pits can detect changes in temperature as slight as 0.003 degrees C. Crotalids use these heat-detecting organs to home in on prey like a heat-seeking missile.
2. Catlike vertical, *elliptical pupils*.
3. A *triangular head* which is distinct from the rest of the body.
4. A single row of *subcaudal scales* (under the tail).

Pit vipers also have heavy bodies and upper fangs which fold back when they aren't biting. And rattlesnakes have rattles, of course, which are thick, interlocking skin segments that accumulate as the snake sheds its skin from time to time. Pit vipers range in size from about a foot and a half (*pygmy rattlesnake*) to over 8 feet (*eastern and western diamondback rattlesnakes*).

Coral snakes are smaller (12 to 48 inches), skinnier snakes, with short, fixed fangs, alternating bands of red, black, yellow or white bands encircling their bodies, black snouts, round pupils, and a double row of subcaudal scales.

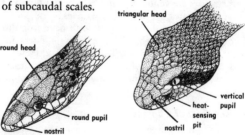

22. a. Nonpoisonous snake.   b. Pit viper.

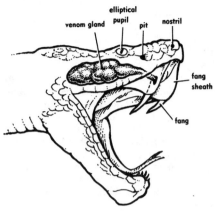

23. *Pit viper identifying marks.*

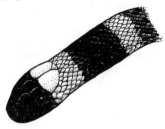

24. *Coral snake.*

Snake Physiology 101

You may not have noticed, but snakes don't have ears. None that you can see, at any rate. But they do have inner ears, and are very sensitive to ground vibrations. And their keen sense of smell derives from their forked tongue, which they use to pick up scents. But their poor vision makes them the Mr. Magoos of the reptile world.

Warm-blooded animals have internal thermostats (humans' are set at 98.6 degrees F). Snakes, being cold-blooded animals, don't have thermostats. Their body temperature fluctuates with the ambient temperature. But, like automobile engines, they have optimal running temperatures. Snakes hum along at 27 to 32 degrees C (81 to 90 degrees F). Below 8 degrees C (46 degrees F), they stop in their tracks, such as they are. And they roast when their temperatures get much above 42 degrees C (108 degrees F). So they sun themselves on rocks on cool days, feed at night during the warm season, and hibernate during the winter.

Snake Eating Habits

Snakes are meat eaters. But they are not aggressive hunters. The rattlesnake's modus operandi is to use its natural camouflage to hide alongside a bunny trail or gopher burrow, wait patiently for a tasty morsel to come within striking distance, and then lunge at it like a fanged rocket. The snake uncoils its body and unhinges its jaws, brings its fangs forward, buries them deep in the animal's body, and injects a lethal dose of venom. The venom paralyzes and starts to digest the shocked critter, who soon finds himself in the unenviable position of being swallowed whole by the snake.

Although their tastes normally run to rabbits or rats, mice, and other rodents, rattlesnakes will bite larger animals or humans when provoked. Most bites suffered by humans occur in the southeastern states and the desert Southwest. And since snakes are most aggressive when they are emerging from or preparing for hibernation, more bites occur in the early summer and early fall.

The Lineup

Here's a rogues' gallery of venomous American snakes:

1. *Cottonmouth.* A semiaquatic snake found in lakes and swamps in the Northeast, and in lakes, ponds, lagoons, and bayous in the Southeast. His mouth has a distinctive white lining. He's a scrappy snake that would make you want to walk on water should you find yourself swimming with him.
2. *Copperhead.* Inhabits meadows, mountains, abandoned buildings in the Northeast, swamps and uplands in the southeastern and central U.S., wooded hills in central Texas. Usually docile, but never trust a snake who can climb trees.
3. *Timber rattlesnake.* Prefers wooded and mountainous areas in the Northeast, wooded rocky hills in the Southeast. Likes to soak up the rays on rocky ledges.
4. *Pygmy rattlesnake.* Prefers swamps, marshes, lakes, and rivers in the Southeast, grasslands in southeast Arizona, New Mexico, and southern

Texas. A nasty little cuss, but his hiss is worse than his bite.

5. *Eastern diamondback rattlesnake*. A big, mean hombre who hangs out in low coastal areas, dry pine woods, and scrub palmetto. He won't run from a fight. The biggest and most dangerous rattlesnake.

6. *Eastern coral snake*. Found in grasslands, dry woods, and along streams in the southeastern states and Texas. Won't bite unless provoked, but then won't let go.

7. *Western (Sonoran) coral snake*. A denizen of the Great Sonoran Desert of Arizona and New Mexico. His potent venom can cause total paralysis.

8. *Massasauga rattlesnake*. Inhabits prairies, dry wooded areas, woodpiles, grasslands, hayfields, and cellars in the central states and prairies in Texas and Arizona. This is a reclusive snake that bites only if cornered.

9. *Prairie rattlesnake*. Favors rock hills and grasslands, open mountain slopes in the central states, and grasslands and hills in the southwestern states. A real snake in the grass.

10. *Sidewinder*. They named a missile after this snake. Hangs out in sandy flats, dunes, and arid, rocky hillsides in southwestern and western deserts. Rests with his body buried in the sand. A real snake in the sand.

11. *Western diamondback rattlesnake*. Found in open and cultivated areas, and near farm buildings in the Southwest and southwestern California. Aggressive, like his cousin, the eastern diamondback.

12. *Northern Pacific rattlesnake*. Lives in semiarid areas to 11,000 feet in northern California, Oregon, and Washington.

13. *Southern Pacific rattlesnake*. Hangs out in semiarid areas in southern California. A laid-back cousin of No. 12.

Modus Operandi

Snakes don't hypnotize their prey, nor do they necessarily hiss or give a warning rattle before they attack. Nor do they have to be coiled to strike. They don't even have to be alive to strike. A primitive reflex enables a severed rattlesnake head to bite for 20 to 60 minutes after decapitation. A 17-year-old boy was envenomated when he impaled his wrist on the fangs of a dried snake head!

Bitter Poison

The potency of a snake's venom and the amount it injects depend on its age, size, the timing of its last meal (it takes three weeks to replenish the venom after a bite), time of year (venom is more concentrated when the snake emerges from hibernation in the spring), and the species. The eastern diamondback, for instance, can inject up to 800 mg of very potent venom, compared with the cottonmouth's 145 mg of moderately potent venom and the copperhead's 40 to 70 mg of mildly toxic venom. The eastern coral snake, on the other hand, only injects 2 to 6 mg of venom, but it gets a lot of bang for the bite. Its venom is 30 times as potent by volume as that of most rattlesnakes.

Putting the Bite on You

Rattlesnake venom is a witch's brew of enzymes that destroy muscle and fat, oxidize amino acids, trigger the release of histamine from cells, cause small blood vessels to leak, rupture red blood cells, and disrupt the normal blood clotting mechanism. But not everyone who is bitten develops an "envenomation syndrome." Around 20 percent of bites are "dry bites" (no venom is injected), and in another 10 percent the snake injects an insignificant amount of venom. If you're not in that happy 30 percent, you've got problems, depending on

1. *Your age and size.* Adults rarely die of snakebite, but children can have severe reactions. The bigger you are, the less vulnerable you are to snake poisoning.
2. *Your health.* Snakebite is especially dangerous in old people, menstruating and pregnant women, and anyone with hypertension, peptic ulcers, diabetes, and bleeding disorders.
3. *Location and depth of the bite.* Snakebites on the head, trunk, and arms are especially dangerous. Injection of venom directly into a blood vessel can put you right into shock.
4. *Duration of the bite.* Rattlesnakes bite and run. Coral snakes don't know when to let go.

Signs and Symptoms of Snakebite

Rattlesnake bites don't hurt much at first. Just a little burning sensation, and you see a fang mark or two, with a little bleeding. But then enzymes in the venom start to liquefy your connective tissues, allowing the venom to spread through the tissues. Other enzymes ravage muscle fibers and fat, denature proteins, rupture cell walls, and lay waste to the landscape, like Sherman marching through Georgia. Within hours, your arm or leg swells up like a balloon, and turns shades of blue and purple rarely seen on this planet. Blebs and blisters pop out all around the bite site. By this time the pain has become intense, you feel weak and nauseated, and you're sweating profusely. As the venom seeps into blood vessels, it ruptures red blood cells and screws up the clotting system. You bleed from every orifice: nose, mouth, rectum, and bladder. By now, several hours after the bite, you're in shock.

Signs and Symptoms of Coral Snake Bites

Coral snake bites are a different story. Their venom contains a neurotoxin similar to the curare that South American Indians used to dab their arrowheads in.

The bite of the eastern coral snake is painless, and produces little swelling and no blisters, discoloration, or necrosis. There may not even be any fang marks. All you feel is a little tingling and muscle twitching at the bite site. You may shrug it off, thinking the snake was nonvenomous. But the neurotoxin works its way through your bloodstream, attaches to your nerves, and starts to exert its grisly effects after a few hours. You may become euphoric, and then get drowsy, or nauseated. Later, you find it hard to swallow, and start drooling. Your vision becomes blurred, your eyelids droop, and then your arms and legs become weak and paralyzed. The gruesome process ends in asphyxiation. But don't lose sleep worrying about the coral snake. Only 40 percent of their bites cause serious envenomation, and fatalities are rare.

Western coral snakes rarely bite humans, and when they do cause only mild neurologic symptoms.

Treatment of Snakebite

It's been said that the only thing you need to treat snakebite is car keys, so you can drive yourself to a hospital for proper care. Many of the traditional measures, such as tourniquets and incision and suctioning, are fraught with danger and of questionable value. Ice doesn't seem to influence the spread of venom in tissues, and you don't need frostbite on top of snakebite. Pressure wraps, although they may delay spread of the venom for a while, do not really prevent swelling, discoloration, and clotting abnormalities and bleeding.

There are a few anecdotal reports of electric shock being used to treat bee stings and snakebites, but this dangerous technique has never been scientifically proven to increase survival.

But the Extractor device, made by Sawyer Products, has been proven to be efficacious. If used within three minutes, it may remove a significant amount of venom.

These are the things that you *should* do after being bitten by a snake:

1. Beat a hasty retreat out of the serpent's striking range (about the length of the snake). He's as anxious to leave the scene of the crime as you are. But if you don't back off, he may bite you again.
2. Keep cool. You can't act rationally if you're excited.
3. If you were bitten by a coral snake, apply a constricting band—but loosely, so that it barely indents the skin. A shoelace or strips of cloth will do the job.
4. Use the Sawyer Extractor if you have one.
5. Splint the bitten extremity, and keep it at heart level. A sling will do for the arm, and you can tie a long splint to the leg. Immobilizing the bitten part minimizes necrosis and delays spread of the venom into the bloodstream. The same logic dictates that you try not to move around too much.
6. Have your buddies take you to a hospital. You can walk to a car if it's less than a 20-minute walk. Otherwise, you should be carried out by litter, horse, or helicopter. If there's going to be a long wait for transportation, let the extremity hang down in a dependent position. If you are alone, start walking. You will probably be able to walk for several hours before severe envenomation symptoms start.
7. Bring the snake with you (if it's dead) so that it can be identified at the hospital.

Here are some tips on snakebite prevention:

1. Stay out of snake country (swamps, caves, deserted mines, and buildings) and avoid rocky crevices and ledges.
2. Watch where you step, sit, and reach. Be careful walking over rocks and fallen logs, and don't reach into holes or bushes. Stay on clear paths when possible.
3. Dress for success. That means knee-high leather boots, long pants, and long-sleeved shirts.
4. Take a friend with you into snake country.

5. The night belongs to the snakes. Nighttime is Miller time for you. Stay in camp.
6. Let sleeping snakes lie. Don't handle a snake unless you're a herpetologist (if you don't know what the word means, you aren't one). Remember, even decapitated snakes can bite.

?❧ LEAPIN' LIZARDS

There are only two species of venomous lizard found in the United States, the Gila monster and its cousin, the Mexican beaded lizard. They are denizens of the Great Sonoran Desert and northwestern Mexico.

These lizards look like giant salamanders. They range in size from 11 to 16 inches, have large, flat heads, massive jaw muscles, short, stubby legs, and long, tubular tails. Their thick skin is a variegated mixture of gray, pink, orange, yellow, and black.

Just the sight of one of these miniature dragons crawling toward you over the sand might kill you. But these charmers also come armed with a venom apparatus consisting of venom glands and nine or ten grooved, lancelike teeth on each side of the lower jaw. Fortunately, the venom rarely causes life-threatening reactions in humans.

The Gila monster is a sluggish-appearing animal. But it sheds that mild image when it goes on the attack. It lunges at its victim, burying its teeth in his flesh. Then it either drops off or starts chewing. If it elects to chew, you're in trouble. Its jaws are powerful, and you may have to use a crowbar to loosen its grip. (And they say that *ticks* are hard to remove!)

A Gila monster bite causes a severe, burning pain that may radiate up and down the limb, as well as a good amount of swelling, bleeding, and bluish discoloration in the bite area. You may break out in a cold sweat, and feel light-headed and nauseated.

Treatment

Treatment is simple, once you've detached yourself from the beast. Copiously irrigate the wound with sterile water, then soak it in antiseptic solution for a few minutes. Make sure you remove any teeth that may have been left in the wound. Then apply a sterile dressing and elevate the part above heart level to minimize swelling. Soak the wound once or twice daily in an antiseptic solution, and be on the lookout for infection. (And make sure your tetanus immunization is up to date.)

15

PLANT DERMATITIS

"Out of this nettle, danger, we pluck this flower, safety."

—SHAKESPEARE,
Henry IV

ल

It's a jungle out there! And I'm not talking about the birds and the beasts. They've learned from hard experience to keep their distance from man. I'm talking about the plant life. Those green things that lie passively about on the forest floor, poking and scratching at you as you walk by. Plants don't have the brains or the decency to get out of your way as an animal does. No respect for the primacy of man. Try to clear them out of your way, and you'll get a hide full of stickers and thorns. Kick them into pulp, and you'll get smeared with sap that will turn your skin into pizza and your eyes into jam.

Don't let their names fool you. A rose by any other name is still poison ivy, oak, or sumac if it gives you a blistering, weeping rash. And daisies, dahlias, and snow-in-the-mountain are every bit as dangerous as their cousins the asthma plant, nose-burn, and crown-of-thorns.

Plants can harm you in one of three ways: by direct mechanical injury, by causing an irritant dermatitis (inflammation of the skin), or by causing an allergic contact dermatitis.

ल MECHANICAL INJURY

Any hunter who has ever ventured into a grouse covert knows about spine and thorns, bristles and briars. A bird ought to feel safe in a place that looks like one of those World War I battlefields. I shudder every time I think of those thornapple trees bristling

136

with spines as long and sharp as bayonets, and those prickle-studded vines strewn along the ground like concertina wire.

You can always pick out a partridge hunter. He's the guy who looks as though he has been mauled by a mountain lion, the one with those hideous scratch marks all over his legs, arms, and face. It's amazing he has any skin left at all after struggling through a no-man's-land teeming with the devil's walking stick and holly, juniper and chokecherry, blackthorn and prickly ash. Working a grouse covert is about as much fun as a date with the Iron Maiden. The seal of the Ruffed Grouse Society ought to be a Purple Heart.

A thorn in the side is better than a thousand barbed hairs in your hand. Cacti and certain weeds and fruits have myriad fine hairs (trichomes) and barbed hairs (glochids) which can be almost impossible to remove once they get under your skin.

Treatment

Those spines, thorns, and bristles rarely cause serious injury. Clean up those scratches with soap and water, and apply Burow's solution compresses to promote healing. Thorns that penetrate the skin should be removed as soon as possible, especially if the entrance wound is over a joint. In that case, you need to watch for signs of joint infection (pain, swelling, and warmth around the joint).

Thorns and bristles that break off under the skin can lead to fleshy growths called *foreign body granulomas*. A week or two after stumbling into a thorn-apple tree you notice a firm, red patch on your arm or leg. Surgery may eventually be required to remove the thorn.

Removing cactus hairs can be like pulling needles out of a haystack. You can try to remove the spines individually with fine forceps, but this can be an exercise in futility. It's easier just to apply a thin film of rubber cement or facial gel over the affected area, let it dry, and pull the hairs out en masse.

?❧ PRIMARY IRRITANTS

There are several groups of plants whose juices contain acids, detergents, and other irritating chemicals that can cause skin irritation. This is not an allergic rash; anyone exposed to the juices of these plants will develop some degree of redness, burning, and itching, depending on the area of the body exposed to the plant. The skin is thick and hard on the palms and soles, and resistant to irritation. The skin on the face, neck, chest, and tops of the hands and feet is thinner and more sensitive to these plants.

Crown-of-thorns, snow-on-the-mountain, candelabra cactus, milk buds, and other members of the spurge family have a milky-white sap that causes a weepy, red, blistery rash. Marsh marigolds, anemones, buttercups, and other members of the buttercup family have a highly irritant oil in their sap that can cause a similar rash.

Nettles have stinging hairs on their leaves that poke into the skin and inject a stream of irritating chemicals that incite a small riot on the skin surface, causing a hivelike reaction. The skin burns and itches intensely for about an hour and remains red for a variable period.

Contact with the mustard seed plant and radishes can lead to blisters.

Treatment

Primary irritant dermatitis is short-lived and doesn't require much in the way of treatment. But make sure you wash the exposed area with soap and water to remove irritant chemicals. Later, you can apply cold Burow's solution compresses, and take an antihistamine to control itching.

?? ALLERGIC PLANT DERMATITIS

Poison ivy or its cohorts in crime—poison oak and poison sumac—grows in every one of the lower 48 states. As a rule, poison ivy is found east of the Rockies, poison oak west of the Rockies, and poison sumac in the Southeast. Poison ivy is rarely found over 4,000 feet or in deserts or rain forests, but grows exuberantly along cool streams and lake shores. It often blankets hillsides that are bathed in sun, but is found only in isolated patches in cool, dry climates. It grows as a deciduous shrub up to six feet in height or as a small tree or vine. Its shiny leaves are arranged in groups of three ("leaves of three, beware of me"), and turn flaming red or reddish-violet in late summer or early fall.

Susceptibility

You may have nothing to fear from poison ivy. Fifty percent of American adults are immune to it. Some people, perhaps 10 to 15 percent of the population, seem to have a natural tolerance to poison ivy. Another 10 to 15 percent are exquisitely sensi-

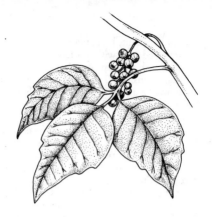

25. *Poison ivy plant.*

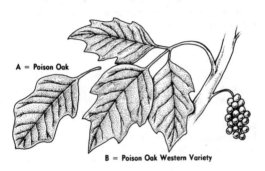

A = Poison Oak

B = Poison Oak Western Variety

26. *a. Poison oak.*
   b. Poison oak, western variety.

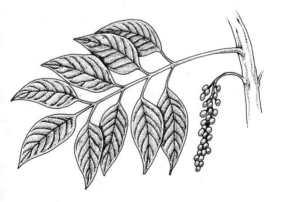

27. *Poison sumac.*

tive to the plant, breaking out in an intensely itchy, blistery, red rash within a few hours of coming into contact with the sap. Another 35 percent are "subclinically sensitive"; they are resistant to poison ivy until middle age, when they suddenly break out in a severe rash after rubbing against the broken leaves or stems of the plants.

No one develops a poison ivy rash the first time he touches the plant. First, the immune system has to be sensitized to *urushiol,* the oil responsible for the reaction. Then, on subsequent exposures, the body recognizes the oil as a foreign substance and mounts a terrific inflammatory response in an effort to destroy it. Repeat exposure maintains the allergic state, but the severity of the allergic reaction tends to diminish with time. And a severe bout of poison ivy dermatitis can actually render a person immune to the oil for a period of time. This is called "hardening."

Urushiol

Urushiol is a sticky, colorless oil that flows through the internal plumbing system of the poison ivy plant year around. When the leaf or stem is broken, the oil is exposed to the air and oxidized, and turns black. (A black stain on the leaves or stem may be the only clue that you are looking at a poison ivy plant after the leaves fall off in the fall.)

The urushiol in poison ivy plants is only slightly different chemically from the urushiol in poison oak and poison sumac plants. If you are sensitive to one of these plants, you are sensitive to all of them. And you may also be sensitive to cashew nut shell oil, mango fruit peels, and Japanese lacquer, all of which contain oils that are chemically similar to urushiol.

Signs and Symptoms

Here is what happens when poison ivy resin comes into contact with sensitized skin: The sap causes immediate primary irritation of the skin, the degree of burning and irritation depending on the amount of oil involved. Meanwhile, the resin quickly penetrates the skin and triggers an allergic reaction. It penetrates thin skin (eyelids, between the fingers and toes, the back of the knees) most rapidly, and these areas may remain highly sensitive to urushiol for up to one year. Even minute amounts of the oil may trigger flare-ups weeks after the rash is healed.

Once the sap of the poison ivy plant touches your skin, you become an allergic time bomb. If the resin isn't washed off within 5 to 10 minutes, it's only a matter of hours (usually 24 to 72) before you break out in a rash. Any area that comes into contact with the resin will react, except the mucous membranes, such as the lips, mouth, and inside of the nose. (There's always the exception that proves the rule. A doctor in Washington reported recently that he developed poison oak urethritis after clearing brush.)

The rash starts off as red, swollen patches, with a few small fluid-filled blisters. As the reaction intensifies, the blisters become larger, and then break down and weep. The whole area becomes covered with an oozing, scaling crust.

The poison ivy rash is one of the itchiest known to man, and it's almost impossible to resist the temptation to scratch it. But this introduces bacteria into the open sores, and secondary bacterial infection is a common problem.

Treatment

The poison ivy rash is self-limited. It usually resolves in 10 to 14 days, no matter what you do. But there are a few things that you can do to ease the intense itching and promote healing.

The most powerful weapon against poison ivy dermatitis is cortisone. But only if it's given early in the course of the illness. A shot of cortisone can be curative if given in the first 24 hours. After that, oral prednisone can be given to tame the inflammation. If you are highly sensitive to poison ivy, ask your physician for a supply of cortisone to take along on wilderness treks.

You can take a more conservative approach to a mild rash that doesn't appear until several days after exposure.

- Cool compresses with Burow's solution relieve the itching and accelerate drying. Do this for 15 minutes 3 or 4 times a day.
- Calamine also helps relieve itching and promotes drying. Apply a layer of it after each session with the cool compresses.
- If large areas of skin are involved, oatmeal baths are helpful. Add a cup of Aveeno oatmeal to the tub, and soak in it for 15 minutes 2 or 3 times a day.
- Aloe vera may aid skin healing. Apply the lotion to the rash twice a day.
- Don't pick at scabs. Soften crusts with moisturizing lotion.

- Antihistamines by mouth will take the edge off the itching, but antihistamine lotions don't help. Anesthetic sprays and lotions not only don't help, they may actually sensitize the skin and aggravate the rash. That can be like pouring gasoline on a fire.
- Hydrocortisone cream is probably helpful only when there is a flare-up after 10 to 14 days, when the rash has almost healed.

Prevention

The obvious thing to do is to avoid the plant. And wear protective clothing, including plastic or rubber boots and gloves. But you can avoid the plant and still get poison ivy dermatitis. Active resin may remain on shoes and tools for years, and urushiol particles on burning poison ivy plants may float into the air on soot and be dispersed over a wide area.

If you are very sensitive to poison ivy, you may want to invest in a bottle of Ivy Shield. This is an organoclay barrier that confers about 95 percent protection to skin exposed to poison ivy.

If you *do* come into contact with poison ivy, wash it off with soap and water immediately. (Water chemically inactivates urushiol.) If your tools or equipment become contaminated, wipe them with a rag soaked in gasoline, kerosene, or some other organic solvent.

A final note: poison ivy is not contagious. You can't give it to another person, and you can't spread it to other parts of your body, unless you have urushiol on your hands.

16

INFECTIOUS DIARRHEA AND FIELD WATER DISINFECTION

"He who drinks a tumbler of London water has literally in his stomach more animated beings than there are men, women, and children on the face of the globe."

—SYDNEY SMITH

❧

Sydney Smith could have been talking about the crystal clear water from almost any wilderness stream in North America. Just because you can see clear to the bottom of the stream bed doesn't mean the water is pure. Chances are, if you could put a drop or two under a microscope, you'd see the same microorganism that Anton van Leeuwenhoek, inventor of the microscope, first saw when he looked at his own stool in 1681: a funny-looking one-celled animal named *Giardia lamblia*. Drink that water without disinfecting it, or even brush your teeth with it, and you may be in for trouble. Within a week or so, your upper small intestine will be carpeted with millions of giardias.

❧ BEAVER FEVER

Giardia is not the only pathogenic microbe cruising the waters of the North American wilderness. It rubs shoulders, or cell walls, with a whole array of gastroenteritis-causing bacteria and viruses, including *Salmonella* and *Shigella* bacteria and the notorious Norwalk virus. But *Giardia* is the number-one waterborne bowel disrupter in the great outdoors. Humans are the major carriers of *Giardia* infection, but many animals carry it, too, and serve as reservoirs of infection. The farther you travel from civi-

143

lization, the less you have to be concerned with waterborne bacteria and viruses, and the more you have to worry about *Giardia*.

You may find it hard to believe that a pristine stream high up in the High Sierra, the Rockies, or the Adirondacks could be fouled with disease-causing parasites, but most such streams are. Here's how it happens: *Giardia* is carried in the small intestine of infected humans, beavers, cows, sheep, and dogs in the mature ("trophozoite") form. Periodically, these trophozoites roll up into hard balls, called "cysts," divided into two, and pass out in the stool. An infected animal may shed millions of cysts each day. These cysts may lay around on the ground or in a lake or stream for two or three months before they are ingested by an unsuspecting animal or human. As the cysts pass through the stomach, they lose their thick outer wall and mature into the active trophozoite form. The trophozoites multiply manyfold, until the walls of the upper small intestine are blanketed with giardias. Through some still undefined mechanism, the giardias cause diarrhea, and the trophozoites are transformed into cysts and pass out in the stool to start the cycle again.

A beaver, deer, or other animal may become infected while foraging downstream from his usual habitat. When he returns to higher elevations, he'll start shedding *Giardia* cysts in his stool. Some of these cysts will eventually be washed into rivulets and brooks, and then into larger streams, until the entire watershed is contaminated.

Mountain streams are prime beaver habitat, and beavers have taken the rap for several large, waterborne *Giardia* epidemics over the years. Dogs, cats, deer, sheep, cattle, and several species of fish, reptiles, and amphibians are also known to be chronic carriers of the disease. But man is chiefly to blame for the spread of *Giardia* to remote wilderness areas. "Backpacker's diarrhea" may be a more fitting sobriquet than "beaver fever."

Signs and Symptoms

Drinking surface water in the wilderness is a roulette game. You may get real sick, you may not get sick at all, or you may only experience a prolonged spell of "acid indigestion," volcanic belching, bloating, flatulence, and diarrhea. But you've got to ask yourself, as you raise that tumbler of ice-cold mountain spring water to your parched, quivering lips, "Am I feeling lucky today?"

Your intestine can become coated with giardias without you realizing that you have become a home for wayward protozoa. You may suffer nothing more distressing then a vague rumbling in your belly and a few loose stools, and you may walk around unwittingly shedding *Giardia* cysts for the next few weeks or months. Or you may feel as though your stomach and intestines were turned inside out and thrown into a washing machine, on the "heavy soil" cycle. You'll start off with explosive, eruptive, camp-disruptive diarrhea. Your stomach will feel like a charcoal pit, and you'll find yourself worshipping at the porcelain throne, or its outdoor equivalent. You'll have foul, jet-propelled flatus (gas produced in the stomach or intestine), fever, a grinding ache in your bones, and plenty of room in your tent as your buddies hightail it for the DMZ. After a few days, a calm will descend over the battlefield, and the belly pain, diarrhea, and flatulence will slowly taper off. That's what "beaver fever" can do to you.

Treatment

It takes an average of nine days for swallowed *Giardia* cysts to sprout into trophozoites, attach to the gut wall, and start beating a tattoo on your GI tract. By that time, you may be back home. On the other hand, you may be hunting elk in a remote area of the Bitterroot Range in Montana. Or you may be trout fishing on Kepimits Lake in western Labrador, your only link with civilization a float plane that won't be back until next week.

Here's what you do if the "GI blues" strike while you're still out in the woods: If *Giardia* is the likely culprit, the ideal treatment is quinacrine (Atabrine) or metronidazole (Flagyl). These antibiotics eradicate *Giardia* from the GI tract in 90 to 95 percent of cases. But it's important that your stool be tested a week or two after treatment to make sure that you are no longer shedding *Giardia* cysts. (If you're venturing into areas where *Giardia* is endemic, especially the Rocky Mountain area, it wouldn't be a bad idea to bring a supply of one of these drugs with you, along with precise instructions from your doctor on how to take it.)

The key to surviving diarrhea, whether it's caused by a virus, bacterium, or *Giardia,* is to avoid dehydration. Take frequent sips of water, juice, weak tea, or other clear liquids. If your fluid losses are large, you'll need to take in 4 or 5 quarts of fluid every 24 hours. Gatorade, ginger ale, root beer, and other sweet drinks are especially good because sugar increases the absorption of water by the bowel. Some foods, such as milk and milk products, caffeine, alcohol, high-fiber foods, and fatty foods, will go through you like the Cannonball Express. But staples such as bananas, cereals, lentils, and potatoes are good sources of calories and nutrients and do not aggravate diarrhea.

You can also mix a batch of the oral rehydration solution recommended by the Center for Disease Control. They suggest that you alternately drink the following mixtures:

glass #1: 8 oz fruit juice, ½ tsp honey or corn syrup, and a pinch of salt
glass #2: 8 oz of treated water and ¼ tsp baking soda

If you are dehydrated, try to drink 8 oz of solution every 30 to 60 minutes (50 to 100 cc/kg in the first 4 to 6 hours, depending on how dehydrated you are).

If, after a few hours of vomiting and diarrhea, you notice that your lips have become parched, your urine dark, and your skin starts to take on the look and feel of parchment paper, then you are well on your way to dehydration. You're running a fluid deficit: there's more going out than coming in. At this point you may benefit from Pepto-Bismol, Donnagel, Imodium, paregoric, codeine, or Lomotil. These are all antidiarrheals or "antimotility agents."

The use of antidiarrheals is controversial. They diminish the force of intestinal contractions and decrease the frequency of bowel movements, relieving you of pain and diarrhea. But theoretically, the *Giardia* or whatever is causing your diarrhea is going to sit in your intestinal tract for a longer period of time, irritating your bowels. On the other hand, if you're losing fluid at an alarming rate, an antidiarrheal may do more good than harm. But be warned: if you continue to have severe diarrhea (more than ten stools a day), persistent vomiting, fever, blood, and mucus in the stool, you need to be evacuated to a hospital. Blood and mucus are not characteristic of giardiasis, and suggest the possibility of colitis, *Salmonella*, or some other bacteria infection, especially if you have fever and chills.

Prevention

Giardia and the other microbes that cause infectious diarrhea are transmitted by the fecal-oral route.

Control their spread by observing these rules of personal hygiene in the wild:

- Bury human waste 12 inches deep at least 100 yards from the nearest water.
- Do not defecate within 40 yards of a lake shore or stream runoff.
- Wash your hands after each bowel movement.
- Do not prepare food if you have diarrhea.
- Rinse cooking utensils and dishes in chlorinated water.

ᔰ WATER DISINFECTION

The only sure cure for giardiasis is to stay away from surface water when you're in the wilderness. But you can have your water and drink it too, *if* you disinfect it first.

The aim in disinfecting water is to remove or destroy the harmful microorganisms in it. What you want is potable water, or water that's safe to drink. It may have a few microorganisms in it, but not any more than your body can easily fight off.

You can disinfect water using physical or chemical methods.

Physical Methods

Whatever method you choose to disinfect water, the process will be more effective if you start with the clearest water available. Cloudy, muddy water is a suspension of silt and clay particles and organic debris that may be contaminated with bacteria and parasitic cysts. You can rely on *sedimentation* to separate out the bigger particles simply by allowing the water to sit for an hour or more. These large particles will settle on the bottom of the container, and you can decant the clear water into another container.

Small particles and chemicals will remain suspended in the decanted water, but you can precipitate them out: Add a three-finger pinch of alum (aluminum sulfate) per gallon of water, stir, and allow the suspension to settle for an hour before you decant it or pour it through a coffee filter or fine-weave cloth. Then disinfect the water using heat or chemical means.

If you don't have alum, you can use baking powder (3 ounces per 5 gallons of water), baking soda (1 ounce per 5 gallons of water), charcoal from a wood fire (2 pounds of charcoal per 5 gallons of water), or fine white ash from a wood fire (2 ounces per 5 gallons of water).

Mechanical water *filters* consist of a screen with pore sizes as small as .2 microns and an activated charcoal element. Micropore filters will remove most bacteria, but not viruses, so the water will have to be either boiled or chemically treated before it is used.

Granular activated charcoal removes bad tastes and odors from water by adsorbing dissolved chemicals. It adsorbs some, but by no means all, viruses and bacteria, so it cannot be relied upon to disinfect water. It's probably most useful for removing chlorine and iodine from water after chemical disinfection.

Heat

If you're not in a hurry, the simplest way to disinfect water is to boil it. *Giardia* cysts are killed immediately in boiling water, and so are most other microorganisms, even at high altitudes.

If you melt snow or ice for drinking water, bring it to a boil just as you would any other water. Chances are, it's just as contaminated as the surface water in the area.

Chemical Disinfection

Chemical warfare was outlawed by the Geneva Convention. But *Giardia,* viruses, and bacteria are still fair game. They are all killed by chemical disinfection with *halogens* (iodine or chlorine). Halogens oxidize the essential cell structures of microorganisms when they are in contact with them in high enough concentration for a sufficient period of time.

Contact time and concentration of halogen are inversely related. The greater the concentration of halogen, the less time is necessary to destroy microorganisms. Conversely, the longer the contact time, the lower the concentration of halogen necessary to disinfect the water. For example, if you double the concentration of halogen, the water will be disinfected in half the time. Or you can halve the concentration of halogen if you simply double the contact time.

The third factor influencing the disinfection reaction is water temperature. When disinfecting cold water, either the contact time or the concentration of halogen has to be doubled to ensure disinfection.

Halogens in high concentrations impart a bad taste to water. The taste of halogen-treated water can be improved by

- Using less halogen and increasing the contact time
- Filtering the water with granular activated charcoal after contact time
- Adding flavoring to the water after contact time
- Using the Sierra Water Purifier (available from 4 in 1 Water Systems, 142 Lincoln Ave., Suite 701, Santa Fe, NM 87501) to chlorinate/dechlorinate the water

HALOGEN DOSES AND TECHNIQUES*

IODINE

Tetraglycine hydroperiodide tablets (EDWGT, Potable Aqua, Globaline)

water conditions	clear	cloudy
warm (>15 degrees C)	1 tab/10 min	2 tabs/10 min
cold	1 tab/30 min	2 tabs/30 min

Solutions

Measure with dropper (1 drop = 0.05 ml).

2% Iodine

water conditions	clear	cloudy
warm	5 drops/15 min	10 drops/30 min
cold	10 drops/30 min *or* 5 drops/60 min	10 drops/60 min

10% Povidone/iodine solution

water conditions	clear	cloudy
warm	8 drops/15 min	16 drops/30 min
cold	16 drops/30 min *or* 8 drops/60 min	16 drops/60 min

Saturated iodine–iodine crystals (Polar Pure)

4 grams of iodine crystals in 2 oz glass bottle. Add water, wait 30 minutes, then decant iodine-saturated water from crystals that remain undissolved, and add this solution to water for disinfection. Remaining crystals may be reused to make new batches of disinfection solution.

* This chart and the one on p. 150 from the Wilderness Medical Society, Position Statements, pp. 14 and 15, 1989.

The dose for saturated solution is calculated at 68–77 degrees F or 20–25 degrees C. If cold solution (37–50 degrees F or 3–10 degrees C) is used, allow it to equilibrate for 60 minutes and increase the dose by 30%.

(One capful from standard 2 oz bottle = 2.5 cc. Doses for Polar Pure are given on the bottle.)

water conditions	clear	cloudy
warm	13 cc/15 min	26 cc/30 min
cold	26 cc/30 min or 13 cc/60 min	26 cc/60 min

CHLORINATION

Halazone tablets

water conditions	clear	cloudy
warm (>15 degrees C)	5 tabs/10 min or 2.5 tabs/30 min	7 tabs/10 min or 5 tabs/30 min
cold	5 tabs/30 min or 2.5 tabs/60 min	7 tabs/30 min or 5 tabs/60 min

Bleach

1%

water conditions	clear	cloudy
warm	10 drops/30 min	20 drops/30 min
cold	10 drops/45 min	20 drops/45 min

4%–6%

water conditions	clear	cloudy
warm	2 drops/30 min	4 drops/30 min
cold	2 drops/45 min	4 drops/45 min

17

MOTION SICKNESS

"The only cure for seasickness is to sit on the shady side of an old brick church in the country."

—English sailor's proverb

ॐ

Bart looked out over the windswept lake and tried to think of something other than the gathering storm in his stomach. He had long since forgotten about salmon. But then, Tom had warned him about Lake Champlain's volatility. When they had left the dock that morning the lake was smooth as glass. Now it looked like the typhoon scene from The Caine Mutiny; *five-foot seas were battering the 27-foot fishing boat, causing it to roll and pitch like a drunken sailor. He ducked into the cuddy cabin and lay down for a while. But that just made him feel worse. He wished he had had the sense to put on one of those patches Tom was wearing behind his ear. His salmon-fishing trip was ruined by seasickness!*

ॐ

Seasickness is the pits. And we are all susceptible to it. Everyone's got a limit to the amount of spinning and turning, dipping and lurching his stomach can take before he heads for the rail. The saltiest Key West, Montauk, and Lake Michigan charter captains have days when the sea is so rough their stomachs flop around like boated salmon. I spent so much time on the water as a boy growing up on Long Island Sound, my parents had to scrape the barnacles off me each fall. I fancied myself a real sea dog, too wise in the ways of the sea to get seasick. But I met my match the summer I went to sea as an ordinary seaman on an oil tanker. A hurricane crossed our path as we steamed past the Outer Banks of North Carolina. My stomach felt as though it were wrapped around the propeller shaft, and I turned a shade of green rarely seen on this planet before the bosun gave me his cure for seasickness: stewed tomatoes, eaten cold with saltines.

Stewed tomatoes cured *my* seasickness. But they may not help *yours*. Besides, medical science in recent years has come up with a number of remedies that are a lot easier to tote around than canned tomatoes. And prevention is the best cure yet, but to prevent motion sickness you need to understand what causes it.

A Balancing Act

Seasickness is an information processing problem. The body has three systems that process raw information about body movement and position and give us a sense of body orientation in space, better known as "balance." Sort of like the way gyroscopes keep rockets upright as they hurtle into space. These are the *visual system,* the system of *body position sensors* (specialized nerve cells in the skin, muscles, and joints that send information to the brain regarding body position), and the *vestibular system.* The latter consists of three semicircular canals and two small bones (otoliths) in each inner ear, as well as their connections to the brain. The semicircular canals sense angular acceleration (spinning motion), while the otoliths sense linear acceleration (straight-ahead motion) as well as gravitational forces. Normally, these three systems work in harmony to keep you on an even keel. The problem comes when you're on a small boat (or in a car or airplane) and you get conflicting information from these different systems. Your eyes may tell you that you're standing still on the deck. (And you are, but the deck isn't. It's rocking and rolling, lurching and heaving, bobbing like a cork on the storm-tossed waters.) But those position sensors in your skin, muscles and joints feel you tensing up, leaning over, bending your legs, moving every which way in an effort to keep your balance on the heaving deck. Meanwhile, your vestibular system is sending a stream of messages to your brain about the different up and down, back and forth, and spinning movements that you are being subjected to. This is a lot of information, and a lot of it is contradictory. Your brain doesn't quite know what to make of all this, so it does the only thing it can do. It orders your stomach to vomit.

Prevention

What distinguishes us from the lower animals is our ability to learn. Our brains are plastic. That is, they are able to assimilate information and use that information to adapt to the environment. If you spend a few days at sea, your brain learns how to handle all that contradictory information the way a teenager handles algebra: it ignores it. That's great, but if you're planning an offshore tuna-fishing trip next week, you probably don't have the time or wherewithal to spend a few days beforehand getting your sea legs.

Nor is that necessary. There is a sea chest full of tricks you can use to ward off motion sickness. Here are a few that have stood the test of time:

- Keep your eye on the horizon or any stationary object, such as a lighthouse, island, or the shoreline. This gives your brain a fixed point to focus on, enabling it to "tune out" most of the other signals coming in from the body position sensors and the vestibular system. Sit in a semireclined position with the head motionless and the eyes straight ahead. Bart, the would-be salmon fisherman, made the cardinal error of lying down in the cabin. He had no fixed points of reference in there, and his seasickness worsened.
- Sit in the center of the boat. There is much less movement there. If you are in an airplane, sit over the wing. In a car, sit in the front seat, or get out of the car and lie on the ground with your eyes open.
- Eat stewed tomatoes and saltines before you set out on the water. Or a cola drink, or whatever you have heard works. If you believe it's going to help, it probably will. I can think of no scientific reason why a full stomach should help, but the placebo effect can be very powerful in this malady in which anxiety and stress play such large roles. Most medical authorities recommend a liquid diet starting a few hours before the trip, with no solids at all until you are back on terra firma. Do what seems to work for *you*.

Medications

Man has been casting about, looking for a magic potion against seasickness since the first caveman set out in a dugout canoe. Almost any concoction you can imagine, everything from creosote to mixtures of horseradish and red herrings, has been swallowed in hopes that it would stave off seasickness. Most of these rotgut combinations don't work, of course. But now, at last, there *is* a magic potion. Well, not a potion, exactly. More like a pill, or a patch.

There are a number of medications that you can take before or during your trip to prevent or treat seasickness. These medications fall into two broad categories: antihistamines and scopolamine. Both antihistamines and scopolamine are thought to prevent motion sickness by inhibiting the flow of nerve impulses from the vestibular system to the brain. Both are effective, but they have different dosages and side effects. Here are the most commonly used preparations:

- Meclizine (Antivert, Bonine). A nonprescription antihistamine that needs to be taken only once every 24 hours, starting 1 hour before embarkation. It causes moderate drowsiness and dry mouth, as do all antihistamines.
- Cyclizine (Marezine). Very similar to meclizine, and also available over-the-counter. It has to be taken every 4 to 6 hours, but it is sometimes effective when meclizine is not.
- Dimenhydrinate (Dramamine). The old stand-by. An over-the-counter antihistamine that is relatively cheap, but it must be taken every 4 hours and causes considerable drowsiness. One advantage is that it comes in liquid form for children.
- Promethazine (Phenergan, Mepergan). This is a prescription antihistamine that is effective in preventing *and* treating motion sickness, but it makes some people very drowsy.
- Scopolamine (Transderm Scop). The latest and (perhaps) greatest. Scopolamine was used in tablet form for years, but caused serious side effects. Now it is available as an ear patch that slowly releases minute quantities of the drug at a steady rate over a period of 3 days. You stick a patch on the skin behind your ear 4 hours before your trip and forget about seasickness for the next 72 hours. It may give you a dry mouth, a dilated pupil on the side where you are wearing the patch, or blurred vision. (Some people who have worn a series of scopolamine patches over a period of days have developed a withdrawal syndrome 48 hours after removing the patch. This consists of nausea, dizziness, sweating, numbness or other strange feelings in the hands and feet, and difficulty concentrating.)

Transderm Scop is an expensive prescription drug, but it is convenient and effective, and the side effects are rarely a problem.

Remember: all these seasickness remedies can cause drowsiness that can impair your ability to drive a boat or a car. This drowsiness is greatly magnified when they are combined with other depressant drugs or alcohol.

18

RABIES, LYME DISEASE, AND OTHER WILDERNESS INFECTIONS

---

*"Some little bug is going to find you some day,
Some little bug will creep behind you some day."*

—ROY ATWELL

➣ RABIES

Rabies. Now there's a word that'll prick up your ears. Make your heart beat a little faster, put a little cotton wool on the roof of your mouth, make you squirm a little. Like AIDS, rabies is synonymous with death. Synonym, nothing. It's become a metaphor for the suffering of the damned. Derived from the Latin word *rabere*, "to rave," it always summons up in my mind the image of a rabid, foaming-at-the-mouth Glenn Ford in that old movie, stalking the streets of a small western town, sending the terrified townspeople running into their houses, where they watch in abject horror as he drops to the dirt and dies in a series of grotesque, jerking spasms.

How Rabies Is Spread

A dangerous myth persists that rabies is a disease primarily of domestic dogs. In Africa, it is. But over the past two decades the incidence of rabies in domestic animals in the United States has declined dramatically, while there has been an upsurge in rabies among wild animals, especially skunks, bats, foxes, raccoons, and bobcats. Of the more than 6,000 reported rabid animals in this country in 1985, only 113 were dogs. On the other hand, 50 percent of skunks and 10 percent of foxes tested in the United States in recent years have been found to carry the rabies virus. Skunks, raccoons, and bats account for 85 percent of animals with rabies in this country.

Wolves, bobcats, coyotes, groundhogs, weasels, woodchucks, cats, horses, and cows can also transmit the disease. Animals *not* associated with rabies include rodents (rats, mice, squirrels, prairie dogs, gerbils, hamsters, and chipmunks), lagomorphs (rabbits and hares), birds, and reptiles.

There are specific geographic distributions for each of these vector species. Skunk rabies is endemic in much of the Midwest. Rabies in raccoons was first reported in Florida in the late 1940s. From there it spread north at the rate of 25 miles a year so that, by 1976, it was endemic in Florida, Georgia, Alabama, and South Carolina. By 1983, 1,608 cases were reported in the Mid-Atlantic States. Only sporadic cases of fox rabies are reported now, and it's largely restricted to Ontario, upstate New York, and Texas. Bat rabies is more widespread, having been reported in most of the nearly 40 species of bats and in all of the continental United States. Eighty-eight percent of all rabid animals in New England are bats.

While there have been only one or two cases of rabies reported in humans in the United States over each of the past few years, the risk of infection is rising as an increasing number of sportsmen hunt and fish in progressively shrinking wildlands.

The rabies virus is deadly efficient. It takes over its host's body to replicate itself, and then drives the animal into a raging fury so that it attacks another animal, where it repeats the cycle. But the diseased animal doesn't have to bite to transmit rabies. All that's required is for infected saliva to come into contact with fresh, open wounds or mucous membranes, such as the lips or inner surfaces of the eyelids. There have been several human rabies cases where the victim was not even aware of being exposed to a rabid animal. And several years ago two spelunkers died of rabies shortly after visiting a bat cave in Texas. Airborne transmission of the virus was suspected after rabies virus was isolated from the air in the cave. There has even been a case where rabies was transmitted in a corneal transplant.

Signs and Symptoms

Here's what happens when an animal (or person) is bitten by a rabid animal: the rabies virus travels up the peripheral nerves to the brain and spinal cord, and then back down the nerves, spreading throughout the body. When the virus is shed in the saliva, the animal becomes infectious. The incubation period can be anywhere from 9 days to more than a year.

The normal range is 20 days in bites to the face to 60 days in bites on the leg.

Following the bite, there is a *prodrome* consisting of fatigue, loss of appetite, headache, fever, cough, sore throat, abdominal pain, nausea, vomiting, and diarrhea. (Sounds like the flu, doesn't it?) After 2 to 10 days, nervous system symptoms appear. The victim complains of anxiety, irritability, insomnia, depression, disorientation, hallucinations, stiff neck, double vision, muscle twitching, sensitivity to light, and he may have seizures. "Furious rabies" follows: the victim will engage in biting, running around aimlessly, and other forms of bizarre behavior. The muscles of the face and throat go into painful spasms whenever he attempts to eat or drink. The mere thought of water will induce these spasms, and he drools to avoid swallowing. Sometimes the mere sight of water is enough to trigger the spasms. This is the well-known "hydrophobia." Fanning or blowing air in his face has the same effect ("aerophobia"). After several hours or days, the rabies lays waste to the nervous system, and the victim becomes paralyzed, lapses into coma, and dies.

There have been only three reported cases of recovery from human rabies. In each case, the victim had received preexposure and/or postexposure prophylaxis and intensive medical care.

You might think, "I don't have to worry about rabies; I wouldn't think of exposing myself to a rabid animal." But here's the hook: classic rabies (foaming at the mouth, unprovoked attacks) is seldom seen in this country. The virus may be excreted in the saliva for a few days before the animal manifests any of the commonly recognized symptoms of rabies. And a rabid animal will attack *without provocation,* even if it doesn't look particularly dangerous.

Prevention

Here's what to do if your *dog* is exposed to rabies: If the animal has been vaccinated against rabies, he should receive a rabies booster shot and be observed for 90 days. If he has *not* been vaccinated, he should be destroyed. (If you are unwilling to do this, the animal *must* be held in strict isolation for six months, and receive the rabies vaccine one month before being released.)

All animal exposures should be reported to the local health department. When possible, the suspected wild animal should be destroyed and the head removed, refrigerated or frozen, and delivered to a veterinarian or health department. They will examine the brain for microscopic evidence of rabies. When *you* are exposed to a wild animal with rabies, destroy the animal and bring the head in for testing. If the animal escapes, check with the local health department. They will make a decision as to whether you should receive postexposure prophylaxis based on a consideration of such factors as the species of animal involved, nature of the exposure (*unprovoked* attacks are highly suggestive of rabies), and whether the animal is available for testing. If the animal is a dog or cat, it should be confined and observed for ten days. If the animal is a stray, it should be destroyed and tested for rabies.

If you are bitten by a rabid animal, you're in trouble. But you won't die like a mad dog unless you ignore the bite. The first thing you should do is wash the wound thoroughly with lots of soap and warm water. Detergents kill the virus, and water flushes it from the wound. You'll need a tetanus booster if it's been more than five years since your last one, and antibiotics to prevent bacterial infection might be a good idea. The sooner you wash the wound, the better. And scrub it up well. This is your only chance to prevent the virus from getting inside those peripheral nerves and traveling up to your brain. You'll have almost no chance of developing rabies if the wound is cleaned within three hours.

There is some good news about rabies. The old series of painful abdominal injections has been replaced by a new vaccine, human diploid cell vaccine (HDCV), that is administered in a series of five shots in the arm or buttock. This vaccine stimulates the body's immune system to produce antibodies to the rabies virus. The shot is virtually painless and is 100 percent effective in preventing rabies when given *before* the exposure. For prophylaxis *after* exposure, HDCV is always given in conjunction with human rabies immune globulin (HRIG). HRIG is serum that contains rabies antibodies. (Antibodies are proteins produced by the body to destroy foreign invaders, including viruses.) A small amount of HRIG is injected directly into the bite and an equal amount injected into the arm or buttock. Both HDCV and HRIG should be given within 24 hours of the exposure.

You have a much better chance of picking the winning lottery ticket than getting rabies. But if you do get rabies, your ticket is punched.

Jack was burning up. The fever had struck out of nowhere, it seemed, and sent a surge of napalm through his veins. Sweat poured out of him in buckets, lacquering his skin and drenching his clothing. He reached down and gingerly touched the tender mat of glands in his groin, wondering if they were in some way connected to the fever.

Jack didn't get the answer to that question until some days later, after he'd staggered out of the woods and driven himself to a hospital. He was shocked when the doctor informed him of his diagnosis: plague.

Jack wasn't lost in a time warp. Now, in the late twentieth century, backpackers and outdoor sportsmen in many parts of the United States are at risk for contracting plague and a number of other exotic infectious diseases. In many wilderness areas rabbits, squirrels, deer, foxes, bear, and other game animals are reservoirs of plague, tularemia, leptospirosis, and various tick-borne illnesses. An apparently healthy animal can carry some mighty virulent microorganisms in his digestive or urinary tract or in the fleas and other parasites that infest his skin. An outdoorsman who is exposed to such an animal is susceptible to a variety of infectious diseases that are unheard of in urban areas. All of these infections are highly treatable, but they are more easily prevented. They key: "know your enemy." Let's take a look at this rogues' gallery of wilderness infections.

Plague

Plague, the infamous "Black Death" which ravaged Europe in the Dark Ages and Asia in this century, continues to smolder in many places around the world, including the southwestern United States. It's a fixture in parts of Arizona, New Mexico, California, Colorado, Utah, Oregon, and Nevada, where it bounces back and forth between wild rodents and their fleas. Deer mice, voles, prairie dogs, chipmunks, ground squirrels, wood rats, rabbits, hares, and marmots all fall plague to plague. Meat-eating animals can get it either by eating one of these infected animals or by being bitten by one of their fleas.

Human plague usually follows the bite of rodent fleas, but can also be transmitted by ticks and body lice, or directly through cuts and abrasions during the process of skinning and dressing infected rabbits. One man got plague after skinning an infected coyote; two others got it after skinning infected bobcats.

Plague bacilli are the marines of the bacterial world. They storm ashore onto an arm or leg and establish a beachhead on the skin. After setting up a local infection, they send armored columns up the lymph channels and overrun the lymph nodes in the groin or armpit, which become swollen and matted together into a tender mass called a *bubo* ("bubonic plague"). From the lymph nodes, assault teams ride the bloodstream to other organs.

In the Dark Ages, plague was synonymous with death, but modern antibiotics make short work of this ancient marauder. Nowadays the infection rarely advances beyond the bubo stage. And you can prevent plague entirely by avoiding contact with susceptible rodents and their fleas; by dousing your dogs liberally with flea powder when in high-risk areas of the West and Southwest; by destroying rodents around lodges or cabins in such endemic areas (but make sure you kill their fleas first, or you'll be their next host); and by taking prophylactic antibiotics when visiting these areas. A vaccine is available and may be a good idea if you live in the rural Southwest.

Tularemia

Plague is tough, but tularemia is no slouch either. This infection comes on like gangbusters, starting with a thermometer-bursting fever and a bone-rattling chill. It's often mistaken for plague, and it causes many of the same symptoms, including skin infections and swollen, tender lymph nodes.

The bad guy here is *Francisella tularensis,* a bacterium transmitted to humans mainly by ticks (dog tick, wood tick, Lone Star tick), deer flies, mosquitoes, and other bloodsucking insects which have taken a blood meal on infected cottontail rabbits, hares, beavers, squirrels, deer, sheep, and other mammals. "Frankie" usually works his way into your blood, if not your heart, through the skin or mucous membranes. He can pass through the skin or the eye when you skin or dress infected animals, especially rabbits, or through the bite or scratch of an infected cat, dog, fox, coyote, or skunk. You can also get tularemia by eating or drinking water or food contaminated with feces or urine from infected animals or fish. Airborne *Francisella* will settle in your lungs and cause pneumonia.

Tularemia is not rare. Several hundred cases are reported each year in the United States. Here's how to avoid becoming a statistic: Wear rubber gloves when skinning rabbits, squirrels, deer, and other mammals, especially in tularemia hot spots such as Arkansas, Missouri, Oklahoma, Texas, and Utah. Cover your clothing and exposed skin with insect repellent, and remove ticks promptly.

Francisella has been recovered from wilderness streams, which is another good reason to disinfect spring, stream, or lake water. And if you like your game cooked rare, you might want to consider leaving it on the fire a little longer.

Leptospirosis

Leptospira icterohaemorrhagiae, the bacterium which causes leptospirosis, is easier to get than it is to spell. Leptospirosis is the common cold of animals, infecting virtually every domestic and wild species the world over. It's been reported in every section of the United States, and up to 50 percent of opossums, foxes, skunks, and raccoons are infected at any given time. What's tricky about this disease is that many infected animals don't become sick, and traipse around in the woods shedding the bacteria in their urine for years. Dogs are notorious for this, and shed leptospiras even after being immunized.

Leptospiras are close cousins of the syphilis bacteria. But leptospirosis it *not* a venereal disease. It's worse than that. This hombre gets into your muscles, giving you body aches the Iron Maiden couldn't match. And your head feels like the top of a ketchup bottle Hulk Hogan is trying to open. Then the fun begins. Fevers and chills like fire and ice. More headaches and muscle aches. The GI tract checks in with nausea and vomiting, gobs of leptospira-infected mucus clog your lungs, causing pneumonia, and you become delirious. After a few days your eyes turn red, and your skin may turn yellow. The leptospiras often invade the central nervous system and cause meningitis and other nervous system disorders.

Leptospirosis is not a common disease, but it's a nasty one, with a mortality rate of about 7 percent. Antibiotics are very effective if started within four days.

The good news about leptospirosis is that you can't get it from the bite of an infected animal. The bad news is, you can get it almost any other way you can imagine. Trappers and hunters may contract leptospirosis by handling diseased animals. But you're more likely to get it by eating or drinking food or water contaminated by the urine of infected animals. You can even get leptospirosis by swimming or wading in contaminated water. The leptospiras enter the body through abraded skin or through the eyes, nose, and mouth. So the key to prevention is to keep food out of the reach of animals, disinfect all drinking water, and wear rubber gloves when skinning animals, especially if you have open sores or cuts on your hands.

?❧ LYME DISEASE AND OTHER TICK-RELATED DISORDERS

Ticks are the commandos of the insect world. The roughest, meanest ticks go on search-and-destroy missions against hunters, fishermen, and backpackers. This is their modus operandi: They load up on bacteria and viruses, climb two or three feet up into a bush, and wait there patiently for their quarry. When an unsuspecting human or animal comes along and brushes against the plant, the tick is catapulted onto his next meal. But he doesn't just eat and run. He drills his syringelike proboscis deep into the skin, gorges himself on blood for a few hours, and injects a slew of disease-causing microorganisms into the bloodstream. The tick's repertoire includes the following:

Lyme Disease

Lyme disease wasn't even discovered until 1975, and now it is the most commonly reported vector-borne disease in the United States. It's caused by infection with *Borrelia burgdorferi*, a close cousin to the whip-tailed bacteria that cause syphilis. The Northeast, upper Midwest, and California and Oregon are Lyme disease hot spots, but it's been reported in most of the lower 48 states as well.

Lyme disease is transmitted by *Ixodes* ticks: the dog tick in the Northeast and Midwest and the Pacific Coast tick in the West. Tick larvae are infected when they feed on deer mice, a reservoir for *Borrelia,* and harbor the Lyme bacteria in their midgut over the winter. In the spring, the larvae transform into nymphs, and the bacteria migrate into the tick's salivary glands. The nymph takes a blood meal on a mouse, deer, dog, or human the following spring or summer, and injects *Borrelia* into its unsuspecting host.

The bacteria then spread outwardly from the bite, causing a large, round, red rash with a clear center. This marks the first of three stages of Lyme disease infection. Fever and tender lymph nodes are also common during this stage. You may feel as though you have the flu.

After a few days or weeks, the rash fades and the Lyme bacteria spread by way of the bloodstream to other parts of the body, including the heart and brain. Symptoms of this second stage include severe headache, rash, irregular heartbeat, and bone and joint pains. If the infection isn't detected and treated, 60 percent of those infected go on to a third stage marked by arthritis of the knee, shoulder, elbow, and other joints.

Lyme disease can be treated very effectively with antibiotics. But it can be hard to diagnose, and many cases go untreated until they reach the second or third stage. Good enough reason to concentrate on preventing tick bites. Wear long-sleeved shirts and long pants when you venture into grassy woodlands during tick season (May through August), and tuck your pants into your socks. You can spray Deet onto your skin and clothing to repel ticks, or just spray your clothing with a repellent containing permethrin. Check yourself carefully once a day for ticks. They prefer warm dark areas, such as the scalp and thighs, so wear light-colored clothing and check these areas extra carefully.

The tick probably has to be attached to the skin for at least 24 hours before it injects Lyme disease bacteria, so prompt removal may prevent infection. Here's the best way to detach the rascal: grasp his head with a pair of fine tweezers and apply steady pressure until he is out. Be careful not to crush him, or the bite wound will become contaminated with his body juices. Then wash the wound with soap and water and apply some antibiotic ointment.

Rocky Mountain Spotted Fever (RMSF)

RMSF does cause a fever and its victims do break out in spots, but it's by no means restricted to the Rocky Mountain area. In fact, it has been reported in all of the continental United States except Maine and Alaska, and is most common in the Middle Atlantic States. The culprit is a rickettsial bacteria which hitches a ride with the wood tick, dog tick, and the lone star tick. "Rick" will get under your skin through the tick's proboscis, but he can also access the bloodstream via abrasions and cuts exposed to tick feces, or when the tick is crushed between the fingers in the process of removal. Ninety-five percent of cases occur between April and September, when ticks are most active and feeding on the blood of dogs, ground squirrels, rabbits, and bear.

RMSF is like a super flu. You start out with a cranium-crunching headache, and then go through the chills and fever, fire and ice routine, muscle aches that would make Mr. T wince, and gut-wrenching nausea and vomiting. After a while, your eyes become sensitive to light, and then you get round, pink spots on your wrists, ankles, palms, and soles. Untreated, RMSF will run its course in about two weeks and carries a mortality rate of 20 to 30 percent. With antibiotics, this figure drops significantly.

Colorado Tick Fever

This is a viral illness transmitted to outdoorsmen by wood ticks throughout most of the western United States and Canada. It's like a mild form of Rocky Mountain spotted fever without the spots. No treatment is necessary, which is a good thing, since none is available.

Tick Paralysis

Some western strains of wood tick secrete a neurotoxin in their saliva that causes paralysis. (This could *really* ruin your elk hunting trip.) Recovery is complete within 48 hours of removing the tick.

19

HIGH-ALTITUDE ILLNESS

"Because it is there."

—GEORGE LEIGH MALLORY,
  when asked why he wanted to climb Mount Everest

George Leigh Mallory was an English mountain climber who disappeared near the summit of Mount Everest in 1929. His fate remains a mystery. He may have become blinded by the snow and toppled off an icy precipice to his death. He may have died of hypothermia. Or he may have succumbed to some form of high-altitude sickness.

You don't have to go to the Himalayas to get high-altitude illness. Most people who rapidly ascend above 8,000 feet develop one or more symptoms of acute mountain sickness. This and the other forms of high-altitude illness can make any high-country venture not only unpleasant but downright dangerous as well.

Here's the problem: Oxygen is the fuel that drives your metabolic machinery. But the machinery starts to sputter when you climb over 1,500 meters (4,900 feet) above sea level and the air gets thinner. As the barometric pressure drops with increasing altitude, oxygen molecules spread out; there are fewer of them in each breath that you take. The oxygen content of the blood drops, so less oxygen is delivered to the tissues.

The body adapts to altitude by

1. Increasing the rate and depth of breathing
2. Increasing the heart rate and the volume of blood that the heart pumps
3. Loosening the chemical bond between oxygen and hemoglobin, so that more oxygen is released to the tissues

Because there is less oxygen in each lungful of air that you breathe, your ability to perform muscular work or exercise progressively diminishes as you ascend to higher altitudes. You have to breathe harder just to satisfy your body's resting requirements for oxygen. Breathing itself becomes a chore. And you develop periodic breathing—waxing and waning cycles of heavy and light breathing interspersed with intervals of no breathing.

This increased work of breathing and periodic breathing wreaks havoc on the sleep cycle. Difficulty falling asleep, frequent awakening, and bizarre dreams are common at altitude. Thus the skier's adage, "ski high, sleep low."

?❧ ACUTE MOUNTAIN SICKNESS

No one knows what the exact incidence of acute mountain sickness is at any given altitude. Anywhere from 12 to 47 percent of people who ascend to heights of 6,000 to 9,800 feet, and up to 55 percent of those who climb to higher elevations, will get it. If you are going to get acute mountain sickness, you'll know within a few hours of ascending to altitude. Whether or not you get it depends upon how high you ascend, how quickly you make the ascent, how much you exert yourself during and after the ascent, how long you stay at high altitude, and your own individual susceptibility to it. Like seasickness, some people seem to be relatively "immune" to mountain sickness. And, just as your body gets used to a heaving deck, you can "acclimatize" yourself to altitudes up to about 17,000 feet.

Insufficient oxygen is the cause of acute mountain sickness, but it's the body's reaction to this deficiency of oxygen that causes the symptoms. Much remains to be learned about this complex disorder, but researchers have shown that insufficient breathing for the conditions, fluid retention, the shift of fluids into the cells, increase in pressure on the brain, and the accumulation of water in the lungs all contribute to the development of acute mountain sickness. Of these, the buildup of pressure on the brain is probably the most important factor.

Symptoms

Mild mountain sickness is like a hangover. It starts with a throbbing headache which is worse at night and on awakening and is aggravated by strenuous exercise, coughing, or bending over. Lassitude,

167

loss of appetite, nausea and vomiting, irritability, and shortness of breath, especially during exertion, follow in short order. You may wake up feeling short of breath at frequent intervals during the night, and develop a dry cough.

Treatment

You can stay put, and the symptoms of mild mountain sickness will resolve in 1 to 3 days. Or you can descend 1,000 feet and get better quickly. Supplemental oxygen helps, if you have it. Limiting your movements also helps. Aspirin, ibuprofen, or acetaminophen will usually relieve the headache of acute mountain sickness. And salt restriction counteracts the body's tendency to retain fluids at altitude.

Acetazolamide increases your respiratory drive and has a number of other effects on body processes. It accelerates acclimatization to high altitude, and can be used both to prevent and to treat acute mountain sickness. Dexamethasone, a cortisone preparation, is also effective in treating acute mountain sickness. However, it has serious side effects, and should be reserved for emergency situations in which descent is impossible, or to help stabilize the victim so that he can be evacuated.

The "Gamow bag" may be the treatment of the future for mountain sickness. It's a plastic bag, large enough to accommodate one or two people, that serves as a sort of "recompression chamber" when it is inflated to higher than ambient atmospheric pressure.

When the victim of mountain sickness starts to stagger, refuses to eat or drink, insists on being left alone, and becomes progressively more confused, disoriented and lethargic, he is suffering from severe mountain sickness and needs to be led back down the mountain right away.

Preventing Mountain Sickness

Here are a few tips on how to avoid mountain sickness. Keep them in mind the next time you go up the hill, unless you own a space suit:

- *Stage your ascent.* Allow yourself time to acclimatize to the thin air at altitude. The key is where you sleep. Your respiratory drive is diminished at night, so that is when your blood oxygen levels fall to their lowest levels. Your first camp should be at 8,000 feet or lower, with subsequent camps at intervals of 1,000 to 2,000 feet. Or you can spend two nights at the same altitude for every 2,000-foot ascent, starting at 10,000 feet. Climb higher during the day, then return to a lower elevation to sleep ("climb high, sleep low").

- *Avoid alcohol,* at least during the first two nights at altitude.
- *Avoid strenuous exercise* until you are acclimatized. Mild exercise probably aids acclimatization.
- A *high-carbohydrate diet* (greater than 70 percent carbohydrates), started a day or two before your climb, will reduce the symptoms of acute mountain sickness by one third.
- *Drug prophylaxis. Acetazolamide* increases ventilation and blood oxygen content, and will prevent acute mountain sickness in most cases. You can take one 500 mg tablet each day or a 250 mg tablet every 8 or 12 hours. If you plan to climb high or rapidly, start taking acetazolamide the same day or one day before you start the ascent.

?? HIGH-ALTITUDE CEREBRAL EDEMA (HACE)

Pressure on the brain causes the headache of acute mountain sickness. When that pressure becomes high enough, sufficient blood can no longer flow into the brain, and the victim is said to be suffering from "high-altitude cerebral edema" (swelling of the brain). One of the most reliable signs of HACE is loss of coordination. The victim can't hold on to a tool or implement, nor can he walk a straight line. He may complain of headache and nausea and may hallucinate or throw a fit. He becomes lethargic, progressively more confused and disoriented, and slips into a stupor or coma.

HACE is treated by immediate descent to a lower elevation, and oxygen and dexamethasone if they are available. HACE is just an extension of acute mountain sickness, so prevention is the same.

?? HIGH-ALTITUDE PULMONARY EDEMA (HAPE)

After a rapid ascent to high altitude, the blood vessels supplying the lung sometimes become "leaky," and the lungs become engorged with fluid. This is called "high-altitude pulmonary edema." It is much more common in young men, and usually develops within the first two to four days after ascending to altitude, often during the second night.

The first signs of HAPE are fatigue, shortness of breath on exertion, weakness, and a dry cough. Severe HAPE is marked by profound weakness, bluish discoloration of the lips and nails, shortness of breath at rest, rapid pulse and breathing rate, a gurgling in the chest, and a cough productive of pink, frothy phlegm.

HAPE is the most common cause of death at high altitude, so it must be recognized while it is still in the mild stage and treated by heading down the hill pronto. A descent of 2,000 to 4,000 feet may be lifesaving. Oxygen, minimizing movement, and keeping warm also help.

Measures that help to prevent acute mountain sickness also help to prevent HAPE.

?• HIGH-ALTITUDE FLATUS EXPULSION (HAFE)

Just as oxygen molecules spread out as atmospheric pressure diminishes, so do intestinal gas molecules. The result is increased intestinal gas and flatus. HAFE has more serious social than medical implications. Immediate descent may be face-saving.

20

DENTAL
EMERGENCIES

"The man with toothache thinks everyone happy whose teeth are sound."

—GEORGE BERNARD SHAW,
Man and Superman

We take our teeth for granted, until they start to hurt. Then, they are more valuable than diamonds. And the intensity of a toothache always seems to vary directly with the distance to a dentist. Consequently, you can expect your worst toothaches, and other dental emergencies, to occur when you are in the wilderness, several days from the trailhead.

Dental emergencies in the wild take many forms. Toothache, lost fillings, bleeding, and broken dentures are just a few of the dental dilemmas that may confront you on the trail. Some of these problems can be prevented by a preemptive visit to your dentist before you set out into the wild. Other problems can't be anticipated. But you can practice crude, and trip-saving, dentistry in the wild if you have a dental first-aid kit. You can purchase a kit or make up your own. It should include the following:

- eugenol (oil of cloves)
- vanilla extract
- tea bags
- zinc oxide powder
- cotton pellets
- cotton rolls
- 2″ × 2″ cotton gauze
- Cavit
- IRM (intermediate restorative material)
- Express Putty
- dental mirror
- dental wax
- #11 scalpel
- small cotton pliers
- toothpicks
- electrical tape
- pen light
- dental broach

Here is a look at some of the dental emergencies you are most likely to run into in the wilderness.

?❧ TOOTHACHE

Teeth are more than little ivory slabs that sit in your mouth and grind food. They are living structures, with a central cavity, called the *pulp,* that contains blood vessels and nerves that supply the outer hard layers of the tooth, the *dentin* and *enamel.* The part of the tooth that extends above the gums (*gingivae*) is called the *crown.* The tapering portion that fits into the socket in the jaw is called the *root.*

The tooth and all its supporting structures are richly supplied with nerve endings. Toothache can be caused by:

Pulpitis

Pulpitis is inflammation of the soft, gelatinous material in the pulp of the tooth. It announces itself with moderate to severe pain, which arises spontaneously or only after the tooth is exposed to heat, cold, or sweets. The pain is generalized, and you may not be able to localize it to any one tooth. You may not even be sure whether it is coming from a top or bottom tooth. But you'll have no doubt which side of your mouth the pain is on. The tooth won't be sensitive to direct pressure, but you can ascertain precisely which tooth is the culprit by applying an ice cube or cold food to each of the teeth on the painful side until you localize the source of the pain.

Most often, pulpitis is secondary to a cavity or a missing filling. Both should be obvious, and both are treatable. First, dry the tooth with a piece of gauze and use a toothpick or a cotton pellet held with cotton pliers to remove as much of the carious material as possible. Then, apply eugenol or vanilla extract to the tooth to deaden the pain. You can make a temporary filling by mixing a small amount of zinc oxide powder with a few drops of eugenol to form a paste. Use a toothpick or the cotton pliers to apply the paste to the tooth. Or you can use Cavit, a premixed filling material. Squeeze a little onto your finger, roll it into a small cone, and apply it to the tooth. Bite it into place, and use a toothpick to shape it. This is only a temporary filling, and you will have to repeat this procedure every few days until you can get to a dentist. Tylenol #3, one or two every 4 hours, may be necessary to relieve nagging toothache.

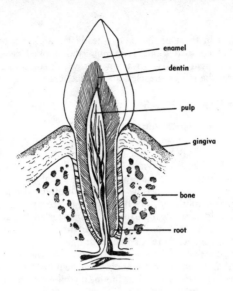

28. Cross section of a tooth

Periapical Periodontitis

This is inflammation of the supporting structures near the root of the tooth. It causes a constant, throbbing pain, and the tooth is sensitive to pressure. The absence of visible swelling over the base of the tooth is what distinguishes periapical periodontitis from infection. It can be caused by trauma or by the leakage of necrotic material from decaying pulp. Minor swelling at the base of the tooth pushes it out a little, so chewing becomes painful. Emergency treatment consists of analgesics, a soft diet, and placing a wad of gauze on the nonaffected side to take some of the pressure off the affected tooth.

Myofascial Pain-Dysfunction (MPD) Syndrome

This is one of those "vicious-cycle" disorders. Stress causes muscle tension, which incites spasm of the muscles in the back of the neck and the muscles of mastication around the jaw, which produces pain, which leads to more stress, which perpetuates the cycle by causing increased muscle tension. An unexpected encounter with a grizzly bear or other tense situations on the trail can cause you to grind or clench your teeth, which can cause an exacerbation of a chronic MPD problem. An acute flare-up will give you pain over the jaw (especially in the area right in front of the ear), a headache, and pain on chewing such foods as granola and smoked meat. Treatment consists of a soft diet, warm compresses over the tender muscles, and analgesics.

ॐ INFECTIONS

Acute Apical Abscess

Bacteria from a cavity spread into the pulp and then through the apex of the tooth into the tooth socket. The usual symptoms are swelling and pain on the cheek side of the jaw. Although apical abscesses are usually preceded by toothache, it often subsides, and the tooth may not be sensitive to pressure, heat, or cold. The ideal treatment is drainage of the abscess, but that may have to wait until you return home, unless there is a dentist or qualified physician in your party. Warm compresses and antibiotics (Pen VK 250 mg every six hours) will help keep the infection under control in the meanwhile. And a soft diet and analgesics help.

Periodontal Abscess

This is a collection of pus between the tooth and the gingiva, usually due to food particle entrapment. The tooth will be sensitive to pressure, but not to heat or cold. And the gingiva will be swollen and tender along the gum line. Treatment consists of numbing the affected area with eugenol or vanilla extract, and then probing along the gum line with a blunt instrument to remove food particles and break up the abscess. Dental flossing, warm salt-water rinses, and antibiotics also help.

Pericoronitis

Pericoronitis is an infection of the gingiva where it covers an emerging wisdom tooth, usually one of the bottom two. It can cause pain on opening the mouth and can mimic strep throat. Repeated biting on the flap of gingiva covering the tooth causes it to swell and become infected. Use eugenol or vanilla extract to numb the area, then remove the flap using a #11 scalpel. Control bleeding by having the patient bite down on a piece of gauze or a wet tea bag for a few minutes (tannic acid in the tea inhibits bleeding). Then have him rinse with warm salt water every two hours, and put him on antibiotics.

Deep Infections

Apical abscesses can spread into the face and

neck, causing diffuse neck and facial swelling and difficulty swallowing or breathing. These are dangerous, life-threatening infections. Start the patient on high doses of Pen VK right away, guard his airway, and evacuate him to a hospital.

?❧ DENTAL TRAUMA

Fractured Tooth

If there is no bleeding from the tooth, the pulp is intact, and no emergency treatment is necessary. If the fracture extends down into the root, remove the loose fragment.

If you see a small amount of blood in the center of the tooth, the pulp is exposed. The tooth will die if it is not attended by a dentist within 48 hours. In the meantime, you can apply a few drops of eugenol, and cap the tooth with IRM (intermediate restorative material, a soothing topical anti-inflammatory dressing) or Cavit.

Loose Teeth

If the tooth is loose but in good position, or looks as though it has been pushed in, leave it alone. If it is out of position, use your fingers to reposition it. Then splint it with Express Putty (3M). After mixing the putty base and catalyst, you have two minutes to mold the material over the loose tooth and two adjoining teeth on each side. Or you can apply dental wax around the tooth to hold it in place.

If the tooth has been knocked out, it should be replaced within 30 minutes or it will probably die. Pick it up by the crown, gently rinse it off, and put it back into the socket. Use dental wax to hold it in place, and give the patient penicillin for a week.

Lost Crown

Find the crown and rinse it off. Apply a few drops of eugenol to the crown, and reposition it onto the tooth. If you get a comfortable fit, remove the crown, apply a little Cavit, and put it back into your mouth. Bite it into place, and use a toothpick to remove excess Cavit. If you can't get a comfortable fit, apply eugenol to the tooth and cover it with dental wax. Save the crown.

Broken Denture

Dry the denture, and then apply a strip of electrical tape to the side of the denture facing the tongue.

21

FOOT CARE IN THE WILD

"*If it is well with your belly, chest and feet, the wealth of kings can give you nothing more.*"

—HORACE

❧

The Roman poet Horace must have had outdoor sportsmen in mind when he penned those lines a couple of millennia ago. Napoleon said, "An army travels on its stomach." And yet it was trench foot as much as hunger which led to his Grande Armée's devastating winter retreat across the Russian steppe. In war as well as in outdoor recreation, nothing will cut a man down faster than aching, blistering, cold, itchy, or wet feet.

Corns, calluses, blisters, athlete's foot, and ingrown toenails are just a few of the characters from the rogues' gallery of foot disorders which can make life thoroughly miserable for a sportsman in the wild. Let's take a look at some of these offenders.

Blisters

Blisters are the result of shear stresses on the skin. When a tight boot rubs across the skin of the feet, the looser superficial layer becomes separated from the less mobile deep layers. The result is the accumulation of fluid in the zones between the skin layers, the familiar blister. You can nip a blister in the bud by applying benzoin spray, Tough Skin, petrolatum, or adhesive tape to sore, red chafed areas. Once a blister forms, the best treatment is to wipe the surface with alcohol, poke a hole in it with a sterile needle (do not remove the skin from the top of the blister, as it protects the underlying skin from infection), and press the fluid out of the blister. Then apply a doughnut pad, or a piece of moleskin with a hole in the

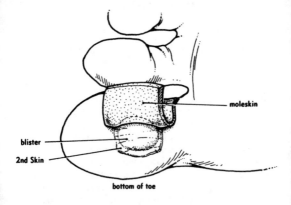

moleskin

blister

2nd Skin

bottom of toe

29. *Cleanse blister with soap and water, then apply 2nd Skin and a layer of moleskin.*

center, directly over the blister, and wash your feet with soap and water daily. The best way to avoid blisters is to wear shoes or boots that fit properly and wear two pairs of socks: a nylon pair under a thicker cotton or wool pair. That way shearing stresses will be redistributed to the interface between the socks.

Calluses

Tight-fitting shoes or deformed feet or toes can produce calluses—thickening of the tough layer of dead cells on the surface of the skin. Calluses are protective, but when they become too thick, blisters will develop at their edges. The best remedy is to keep them trimmed with a callus file. When calluses return, apply a pad or adhesive tape over prominent bones where calluses form. If the problem is a crooked heel, a heel cup may be the answer; it spreads the force of heel strike over a wide area of skin. The last resort is a new pair of boots.

Corns

Have you ever had painful little volcano-shaped craters between your fourth and fifth toes? These are corns, a type of callus. They are painful because the skin at the bottom of these craters is perpetually bathed in perspiration, which causes it to become very thin and sensitive to pressure. These calluses are usually secondary to a prominence on the outer surface of the fourth toe. The best treatment is to wear wider boots. A wisp of cotton between the toes soaks up the perspiration and decreases pressure on the skin. Corn pads are good, too.

Ingrown Toenails

Tight boots can also cause ingrown toenails. The thick, rigid edge of the nail of the big toe digs into the adjoining skin, producing redness, irritation, swelling, and "weeping" as the inflamed skin secretes fluid. There are a number of ways to deal with ingrown toenails. First, cut a "V" in the middle of the nail to make it more flexible. Then fold a small sheet of aluminum foil until it's the size of a match head and insert it under the corner of the nail where it's digging into the skin. Place a wisp of cotton along the nail to keep the area dry, and keep the foot elevated as much as possible. If these conservative measures don't work, or infection develops, see your doctor.

Athlete's Foot

After a day or two of walking the ridges for spring turkey, or stalking Rocky Mountain elk over miles of rough terrain, your feet can get downright grungy with accumulated sweat. The heat and moisture inside your boots encourage growth of *Trichophyton*, the fungus that causes athlete's foot. Scaling, red, intensely itchy areas, with vesicles and fissuring between the toes, are characteristic of this condition (which is *not* easily transmitted from person to person, contrary to popular belief). The key to prevention and cure is to eliminate heat and perspiration. Wear shoes and light cotton socks that allow for adequate ventilation. Wash and gently dry the feet every day, if possible, and apply tolnaftate (Tinactin) liquid to infected areas twice daily. Sprinkle an antifungal powder containing tolnaftate or undecylenic acid (Breeze Mist Foot Powder) between the toes and into the socks every morning. The powder will soak up moisture and destroy the fungus before it can establish a toehold on your feet.

General George Patton was right on target when he said, "It's a hell of a lot more important to keep your feet clean than it is to brush your teeth! You do not walk on your teeth! You use your feet all the time to get at the enemy. Keep your feet clean."

22

WILDERNESS SURVIVAL

"We do not choose survival as a value; it chooses us."

—B. F. Skinner

Merchant seaman Poon Lim survived 133 days on a raft in the Atlantic Ocean during World War II. When your world is a raft bobbing on the sea, your needs are stripped to the basics: oxygen, water, enough heat to maintain a core temperature of around 99 degrees, and sufficient food to keep the metabolic furnace running.

If the spirit is willing, a human being will find a way to survive under the most adverse conditions. While Poon Lim was drifting across the Atlantic, German soldiers on the Eastern Front sought refuge from the brutal cold inside the bellies of disemboweled horses. Greenland Eskimos have been known to crawl inside their dogs to keep warm, and even eat them when it's a matter of survival. Shipwrecked sailors have been known to take sustenance from every manner of flying and crawling beast, from roaches to rats to snakes. Members of an Uruguayan rugby team that crashed high in the Andes Mountains of Chile some years ago survived by resorting to cannibalism.

COLD-WEATHER SURVIVAL

In Chapter 8 we looked at the ways in which the body attempts to maintain a core temperature within the narrow limits of 95 to 100 degrees. Heat can be generated quickly by any form of muscular exercise. And metabolic heat production can be increased by eating food with a high SDA (specific dynamic action); this is the increase in the body's basal metabolic rate that results from eating various kinds of foods. Proteins have the highest SDA, but carbohydrates are metabolized more easily than fats and proteins and heat the body more rapidly. It is important to eat frequently, at least every two hours, when outside in cold weather. Alcohol and tobacco, which predispose to hypothermia and frostbite, should be banished from the trail.

Shelter

No matter how warmly you are dressed, you can't survive outside indefinitely in the cold. Eventually, you are going to need to find or construct a shelter.

The key to preserving body heat is to eliminate the wind-chill factor by finding a windbreak of some kind. You can ride out a snow squall in the mouth of a cave, in a tree hollow, under a cliff overhang, in a lean-to, or on the lee side of a large rock or tree (a "tree well"). You can be reasonably comfortable in such a shelter if you build a fire, and amplify its heat by building a barrier wall of logs or stones on its far side to reflect the fire's radiant energy back onto you. (But make sure that there are no snow-laden branches overhead. The snow will inevitably end up on the fire.)

You can enhance any shelter by building a windbreak of snowblocks or boughs about two to three feet high and two to three feet to windward of the shelter. If the windbreak is placed much farther away from the shelter, drifting snow will bury the shelter.

Building a Snow Cave

Snow is one of the best insulating materials, which makes it a good construction material for a temporary shelter. You can build a *snow cave* by burrowing mole-fashion into the side of a snowbank. Slant the entrance tunnel upward, and excavate just enough snow to create a space large enough to kneel and stretch out in a sleeping bag. The sleeping platform should be elevated 18 inches off the floor and covered with boughs for insulation. Drill a ventilation hole through the roof, and one in the snowblock used as a door. If you keep the cave small, you can heat it a few degrees with a candle.

Building a Snow Trench

Digging a snow cave can be a time-consuming process, and you'll be drenched with sweat by the time you are done. The sweat will accelerate evaporative heat loss from your body, and that's obviously counterproductive. A *snow trench* may be a better idea. It's easier to build and doesn't require as much snow. You can construct an emergency shelter for two people in twenty minutes. Use a ski or pot to scoop out a pit three feet deep, four feet wide, and eight feet long at the surface. Then, undermine the edges so that the trench is eight feet wide and ten feet long at the bottom. Then, lay skis, ski poles, or long branches width-wise across the top of the trench, cover this frame with a tarp or evergreen boughs, and pile snow or rocks along the edges of the tarp to hold it in place. If you leave one end of the trench open, you can build a fire at that end. If you have a propane or sterno stove, you can completely enclose the top of the trench, leaving only a narrow entrance and a six-inch ventilation hole at one end. Whichever way you do it, don't let the temperature inside get above freezing, or your shelter will melt and you'll have to contend with water in your sleeping bag.

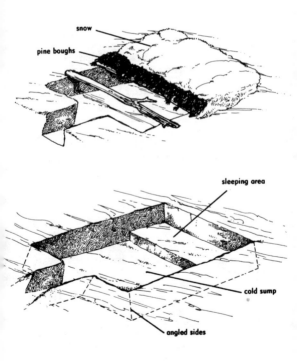

30. Building a snow trench with a bed platform.

Starting a Fire

Every man prides himself on being an expert fire starter, but starting a fire in a raging blizzard is no mean feat. Here's one surefire technique: gather some of the small, dead lower branches from evergreen trees, as well as a few pieces of birch bark, dry leaves or grass, plant stems, or other tinder. Clear a space on the ground, out of the wind, and arrange the twigs as a lean-to across a log or in wigwam fashion. (If you can't find dry twigs, whittle a pile of shavings off a stick.) Ignite the tinder, and apply kindling as the fire grows. Split soft woods ignite most easily and make the best kindling.

Add fuel slowly so that you don't smother the fire. After you get a good, hot fire going with soft woods, switch to hard wood fuel. It burns slowly and leaves lasting coals. Keep the fire small to conserve wood, and maintain a healthy supply of fuel by collecting several times more than you think you will need.

Starting a Fire Without Matches. You can try rubbing two sticks together, but there are easier ways to start a fire:

- Use the lens of a camera, binoculars, telescopic sight, or flashlight to focus sunlight on a pile of tinder.
- Use your knife or any piece of hard steel to strike sparks on a piece of flint, quartz, or pyrite. You can use charred rags, bird down, pulverized bark, or dry moss for tinder.
- Attach wires to the positive and negative ends of two C or D batteries in tandem, and scratch the ends together to create a spark.

?❧ FOOD

In Louis L'Amour's novel *Last of the Breed,* American fighter pilot Joe Mack escapes from a Soviet prison camp and disappears into the Siberian wilderness. He relies on the survival lore he learned from his Sioux Indian grandfather to live off the land while he treks across thousands of miles of forbidding terrain with the KGB in hot pursuit. He traps small animals for food, fashions moccasins and clothing from their pelts, and supplements his diet with berries, herbs, and nuts he gathers in the woods.

The average man needs to take in 3,000 calories a day, twice that much if he is exercising vigorously in the cold. If you're stranded in the wilderness, and don't have the survival savvy of a Joe Mack, here are a few guidelines as to what is edible and what is not:

- Test any food before eating large amounts of it. If it hasn't made you sick after 4 or 5 hours, it's probably safe to eat.
- These parts of wild plants are edible: nuts; grass seeds; the roots and young curled fronds of ferns; berries (except water hemlock and baneberry); the bark of aspen, cottonwood, birch, willow, and the inner bark of scotch and lodgepole pine; leaves of mountain sorrel, young willows, and fireweed (if boiled); aspen and poplar buds, spruce and tamarack shoots.
- Birds' eggs, all land mammals, birds, crustaceans, mollusks, and insects are edible. Some amphibians (not toads) and reptiles are safe to eat. Fish are generally edible, except for Pacific reef fish and blowfish and other "puffers."
- Cook all wild foods except fruits and berries.
- Some lichen are edible. Boil or roast reindeer moss, boil Iceland moss for one hour, and dry and boil rock tripe.
- Steer clear of mushrooms, buttercups, and plants with a milky sap.

Edible nuts are the most nourishing forest foods. Buds are also good, and stems are excellent sources of sugars, starches, and oils. Leaves can be made more palatable by leaching. Boil them until the bitter taste is removed.

?• WATER

Do you realize that you've been lugging around 40 liters of water most of your life? That's how much water there is in the average 70 kg man's body. Each of your 100 trillion cells is a miniature ocean, and virtually every tissue in your body is bathed in a salt-water solution. You can survive without food for weeks, but you can only make it for a few days without water. When you go without food for a while, your body is able to mobilize energy stored as fat and sugar compounds in the muscles and liver. It can even convert muscle and other tissues into energy if the situation gets desperate enough.

But humans can't store water in humps the way camels do. Water that is absorbed through the intestine goes immediately into the cells, the extracellular fluid, the blood plasma, or one of the other body fluids. Each day approximately 1,400 ml of water is lost in the urine, 100 ml in the sweat, 300 ml in the stool, and 700 ml by evaporation through the lungs or skin. In order to keep from getting dehydrated, you need a constant supply of water, 2,400 ml a day on average. Six hundred ml of water is produced by the metabolism of food, so you need to drink a minimum of 1,800 ml. In a hot climate or during vigorous exercise, your water requirements increase dramatically. After about 36 hours at a high altitude, your kidneys start working overtime, so you should drink at least 3 or 4 liters of water a day when you are above 8,000 feet.

Don't let thirst be your guide to your water requirements. The thirst center in your brain isn't stimulated until your cells become dehydrated. Keep ahead of the game by drinking liberally whenever you have the opportunity. And keep your canteen full.

Avoid eating snow. It takes too much of your body's energy to melt, and you don't know what fungi or bacteria are on it. Be especially wary of pink or stale snow. If you are going to melt snow on a fire or stove, or on a dark sheet in the sun, you'll get more water out of hard, packed snow or ice than freshly fallen powder snow.

Drinking urine or seawater is taboo. Seawater has three to four times the concentration of salts as body fluids, and even small amounts of it can cause dangerous elevations of sodium, potassium, and magnesium in the blood. Urine is loaded with metabolic waste products and will poison you.

Solar Still

If you have a plastic sheet, you can make a solar still and reprocess urine or water from vegetation. Scoop out a hole two feet deep by three feet across and put a clean pail or container in the center of the hole. Pull up some grass or other vegetation and scatter it around the bottom of the hole. Or put a bottle filled with urine in the hole. Then stretch the plastic sheet across it, securing it with logs or rocks. Water from the grass or urine will condense on the undersurface of the plastic sheet, and roll down to the center and into the pail.

Vegetation Still

Take a large bag (a clear one, preferably) and fill it with vegetation. Then inflate the bag, tie off the top, and place the bag in the sun. After a few hours, water from the vegetation will condense and collect in the bottom of the bag.

You can obtain at least a little water by squeezing any freshwater fish and many plants. Small streams that run at right angles to the drainage system can be considered relatively safe to drink from. But boil the water first to be safe.

?❧ DESERT SURVIVAL

A third of the world's land surface is covered by desert. Half of this is the cold desert of the polar regions. The other half is hot, arid wasteland populated only by a few plant and animal species especially adapted to this harsh environment.

Deserts are not only hot by day (a thermometer-bursting 136.4 degrees F in the shade at El Azizia, Libya, on September 13, 1922) but surprisingly cool at night. Sand and rocks warm up quickly during the day, but release their heat quickly at night. Nor is there much moisture in the desert air to retain heat, so the mercury can plummet 35 to 45 degrees after sunset.

The desert floor can get hot enough (185 degrees) to burn your shod feet. But there are other things going on that will keep you hopping—like flash floods, dust storms, and rattlesnakes. Not to mention the sharp rocks and thorns strewn along the ground. And sunburn is an omnipresent danger.

When it comes to desert attire, you can tear a page from the Bedouin's book. Their light-colored, loose-flowing robes protect them from sunburn and allow for adequate ventilation, while insulating them from the chill night air. And cotton is the material of choice in the desert. Its low insulating value and high wicking action allow for rapid heat dissipation and sweat evaporation in hot weather. An SPF-15 or greater sunscreen, good-quality sunglasses, and a wide-brimmed hat with a foreign-legion-style flap in the back will complete your protection against sunburn and sun glare. (If you don't have a hat, you can fashion an Arab burnoose out of a T-shirt or a piece of cloth.)

Shelter

You won't survive long without water in the desert, so if your canteen runs dry, you're going to have to strictly conserve body fluids. Lay low during the day and travel at night when it's cool and you are less likely to sweat. The hottest place in the desert is the top few inches of the ground and the air a foot or so above the ground. If you scoop away a layer of sand, you'll find the ground surprisingly cool. You can look for a rock overhang or use a plastic sheet or tarp to rig up a sun screen. Or you can look for a natural shelter or stay in your stranded vehicle. But don't bed down in an arroyo or gully unless you want to get washed away in a flash flood.

Food

There's food all around you in the desert, but you have to look for it. Any crawling, leaping, or flying creature is fair game, including snakes, insects, rats, and lizards. Most vegetation is edible, including cactus fruits, wild cherries, wild currants, wild celery, piñon nuts, the soft parts of grass stalks, and seeds.

Water

All roads lead to water in the desert. At least all animal trails do. Watch which way the critters are heading at dawn and dusk, and follow them. You won't go wrong. But beware of any pool that doesn't have animal tracks and droppings.

You can collect dew from leaves, flowers, or any cold surface. The flowers and fruits of plants, especially the fruit of the saguaro cactus, are loaded with water after a rainfall. After a heavy rainfall, look for water in the hollows of rock formations. And look for springs at the foot of cliffs or in gullies. Or try digging for water in the outer bends of dried stream beds.

23

THE WILDERNESS MEDICAL KIT

"It is thrifty to prepare today for the wants of tomorrow."

—AESOP,
"The Ant and the Grasshopper"

"Preparation is the key to victory."

—GENERAL DOUGLAS MACARTHUR

₂♥

What's the first thing you look at every morning, after you stumble sleepy-eyed into the bathroom? Your mug in the mirror. And what's behind that grisly visage? Why, the medicine cabinet, of course. It's right in front of your face, conveniently situated so that you don't forget to take your medicines. But what do you do when you're camped out on the banks of the Snake River in Idaho or bivouacked on some Rocky Mountain peak during elk season? Do you pack all your medicines in a neatly organized satchel, or do you just throw them all into an old sock?

It seems that you never need half that stuff in your medicine cabinet until you're out in the woods somewhere, fifty miles of bad road between you and the nearest drugstore. Then you'd trade your sleeping bag for a bottle of calamine lotion for that poison ivy rash, or a couple of aspirin for that headache. And you'd pay a king's ransom for a bottle of Donnagel to ease those stomach cramps and diarrhea.

It would be nice if you could just pull that medicine cabinet out of the wall and throw it in the back of the truck along with the rest of your gear. But it would be easier to make up a medical kit, a sort of portable medicine cabinet, containing all the medical supplies you will need for emergencies in the field. We are not talking about a Mobile Army Service Hospital, but a kit that you can tote around in a tackle box or a small canvas satchel. And you can make up a smaller kit-within-a-kit to stick in your fishing vest or your back pocket when you go afield.

The key to putting together a useful kit is organization. If you just go out to the drugstore, buy the items I have listed, and cram it all into an old sack, you might as well call it Pandora's box. Let's stay organized by grouping the supplies as follows:

?❧ WOUND CARE MATERIALS

bar soap
antiseptic solution, 4 oz bottle
triple antibiotic ointment, 1 oz tube
12 Adaptic dressings, 3″ × 3″
24 sterile dressing pads, 4″ × 4″
4 Kerlix or Kling roll bandages, 4″ × 5 yd
3 Surgipads, 8″ × 10″, or ABD pads, 8″ × 8″
1 roll waterproof adhesive tape, 1″ × 5 yd
8 Bioclusive or Tegaderm transparent dressings, 2″ × 3″ or 3″ × 3″
Spenco 2nd Skin
50 bandage strips (Band-Aids), 1″ × 3″
Surgical staples (Precise Five-shot, 3M)
10 skin closure strips, ¼″ × 3″
10 skin closure strips, ½″ × 3″
1 compound benzoin tincture, 2 oz
4 sterile eye pads

Bar soap (Dial, Ivory) is fine for daily cleansing of abrasions and superficial burns.

Antiseptic solution. Povidone-iodine 7.5% (Betadine), benzalkonium chloride, and chlorhexidine (Hibiclens) are three good ones.

Triple antibiotic ointment (Neosporin, bacitracin). Apply a small amount to a wound before covering it with a dressing.

Adaptic pads. These are nonadherent mesh dressings that prevent the bandage from sticking to the wound.

Sterile dressing pads. 4-ply pads with a wicking action that absorbs blood and other fluids from wounds. Good for cleaning wounds as well.

Kling and Kerlix roll bandages. Stretchy gauze rolls for bandaging and securing splints.

Surgipads, ABD pads. You can use these big, bulky bandages to apply pressure to large, bleeding wounds and to cover burns.

Bioclusive or *Tegaderm transparent dressings*. Space-age technology in a wound dressing, they seal out water and dust, but not air. Ideal dressing for blisters, abrasions, and small cuts that are not bleeding.

Spenco 2nd Skin is a hydrogel (96% water, 4% polyethylene oxide) that's a great field dressing for open blisters and burns. It soaks up fluids and reduces pain and friction.

Skin closure strips. Butterflies (Johnson & Johnson), Steri-Strips (3M), Curi-strips (Kendall), and Coverstrip Closures (Beiersdorf). These sterile strips can often be used in lieu of stitches to close cuts. They'll stay on longer if you apply *tincture of benzoin* to the skin on either side of the wound and let it dry until it becomes "sticky." (*Warning:* Benzoin is an organic solvent—don't let it come into contact with the wound itself.) *Caution:* Skin closures are best reserved for "clean," relatively superficial wounds. Deep, jagged lacerations are best treated in a medical facility.

Dressings and bandages should be stored in a watertight plastic container to ensure that they don't get wet.

Medicines

100 aspirin, acetaminophen, or ibuprofen tablets
10 dimenthydrinate (Dramamine) 50 mg tablets or 10 meclizine 25 mg tablets
20 diphenhydramine (Benadryl) 25 mg tablets
Donnagel, 4 oz
30 Lomotil tablets
10 Phenergan suppositories, 50 mg
30 Tylenol No. 3
40 Pen VK 250 mg tablets
20 Duricef 500 mg capsules
30 acetazolamide 250 mg tablets
16 Decadron 4 mg tablets
4 Transderm Scop discs
Maalox, Mylanta, or other antacid, 5 oz
calamine or Caladryl lotion, 8 oz
12 Domeboro tabs
sulfacetamide 10% ophthalmic drops, 10 cc
tetrahydrozoline eye drops 0.05%, ½ oz
miconazole cream 2%, ½ oz
hydrocortisone 0.5% cream, 1 oz
Solarcaine first-aid lotion, 3 oz
sunscreen SPF 15 or greater, 8 oz
zinc oxide, 1 oz
Cavit, 7 gram tube

Personal Medications

Dramamine is the old standby for motion sickness. *Meclizine* is also very effective and can be taken once a day.

Diphenhydramine (Benadryl) should always be on hand for allergic reactions and to control severe itching from poison ivy or other causes. It's good for nausea and sleeplessness too.

Donnagel is liquid gold when diarrhea and cramps strike in the deep woods. *Lomotil* is a more potent prescription antidiarrheal.

Phenergan suppositories will put the stops to nausea and vomiting.

Tylenol No. 3 is a potent analgesic, but is also good for coughs and diarrhea. Each tablet contains 300 mg of acetaminophen and 30 mg of codeine.

Pen VK is penicillin. This is the drug of choice for dental infections and strep throat. *Duricef* is effective against staph bacteria and is effective in treating wound infections and other soft-tissue infections.

Acetazolamide and *Decadron* are useful in treating mountain sickness.

Transderm Scop patches can prevent motion sickness.

Calamine drys weeping, itching poison ivy rashes. One or two *Domeboro* tablets can be added to a pint of water to make Burow's solution, an astringent, drying solution.

Tetrahydrozoline drops (Visine a.c., others) soothe eyes reddened by smoke or sun.

Miconazole cream (Micatin and others) cures athlete's foot.

Cavit. A dental paste for emergency repair of lost crowns and fillings.

Zinc oxide is a physical sunblock.

≈ MISCELLANEOUS

2 instant cold packs
2 elastic bandages, 3″ × 6″
rubber tourniquet, 1″ × 24″
bee sting allergy kit (Anakit)
bulb irrigating syringe, 60 cc
triangular bandage
6 safety pins
2 tongue blades
scissors
tweezers
scalpel handle and #11 blades

pliers
snake suction device
spare eyeglasses
signal mirror
magnifying glass
penlight flashlight
waterproof matches
Sam splint

Elastic bandages (Ace). Are good for wrapping sprains and applying compression to large, bleeding wounds.

A *tourniquet* can save your life when severe bleeding cannot be controlled by direct pressure. (*Caution:* A tourniquet can cause irreparable harm to blood vessels and nerves. Loosen it at least every two hours, and remove it as soon as the bleeding can be controlled by other means.)

Insect sting kits (Ana-Kit) contain a prefilled syringe of adrenaline and antihistamine tablets (chlorpheniramine) for self-treatment of severe insect sting reactions. If you're allergic to bees, don't leave home without one.

Triangular bandage. A large muslin bandage can be used as a shoulder sling, turban bandage for head wounds, or to secure splints to fractured extremities.

Safety pins have many uses: securing slings and splints, closing large wounds, holding the tongue out of the back of the throat when the jaw is badly broken.

Tongue blades (or depressors) make good splints for fractured fingers.

Needlenose pliers. For removing fish hooks, of course.

The Extractor is a snake venom suctioning device available from Sawyer Products, P.O. Box 188, Safety Harbor, FL 34695 ($14.95).

Dental first aid kit. See Chapter 20.

This is a comprehensive list. How many of these items you actually need in your kit depends on the number of people in your group, the level of medical expertise in the group, the expected risk of injury or illness during the trek, the duration of the trek, and the maximum distance you will be from medical help at any point during the trek. You will have to ask your doctor for prescriptions for the items not available over the counter.

The equipment in the kit should be consistent with the skills of the most medically sophisticated member of the group. There is no point in packing hemostats and scalpels if no member of the group has ever seen the inside of an operating room. On the other hand, a qualified physician would probably like to see some intravenous solutions and injectable medications included in the kit.

The kit as described would be a load to lug around on a long trek. One way around that problem is to have each member of the group carry his or her own personal medical medications, as well as a portion of the medical kit.

?* A KIT-WITHIN-A-KIT

The President is followed wherever he goes by a naval officer lugging a "black box" containing nuclear weapons codes. Unless you have someone like that to carry around your medical kit, you'll probably elect to leave it in camp when you set out upcountry each morning. But you *can* pack a small first-aid kit. Store the following items in a small, waterproof case in your pocket or in a "fanny pack":

antiseptic solution, 1 oz
6 adhesive bandage strips
4 skin closure strips
4 sterile gauze dressings, 4" × 4"
waterproof adhesive tape, ½"
waterproof matches
triangular bandage
aspiring/ibuprofen/acetaminophen tablets
snake suction device (if you are in snake country)

It is also a good idea to carry the following items on your person at all times:

Identification, including a list of medical problems, allergies, and medications
Bandana (doubles as a bandage or sling)
Coins for telephone
Cord
Swiss Army Knife

INDEX

ABCs (airway, breathing and circulation):
  in CPR, 15–16
  in drowning, 114
  for head and neck injuries, 48–49
  for lightning injury, 105
  for shock, 10–11
abdomen, 61–62
  blunt injuries to, 61–62
  penetrating injuries to, 62
ABD pads, 188
abrasions, 27
  corneal, 63–65
abscesses, dental, 174
acetazolamide, 168, 190
acute apical abscess, 174
Adaptic pads, 188
AIDS, 156
airway:
  in choking, 12
  in CPR, 15
  in drowning, 114
  head and neck injuries and, 48
  lightning injury and, 105
  in shock, 10
alcohol:
  drowning caused by, 109
  hypothermia caused by, 74, 79
allergic plant dermatitis, 138–42
altitude, solar injuries related to, 89–90
aluminum, as electrical conductor, 107
amputations, 46
ankles, 41–42
antidiarrheals, 146
antiseptic solutions, 188
ants, 123, 124
apical abscess, acute, 174
arc burns, 33
aspiration, 108, 110–11
  of brackish water, 111
  of fresh water, 110
  of seawater, 110–11
athlete's foot, 178
atmospheric conditions, solar injuries related to, 89–90
avulsions, skin, 24–25
Back injuries, 39–40
ball lightning, 101
bandages, 188, 191

basal cell carcinoma, 91
basics, 7–17
    choking and, 11–14
    CPR and, 14–17
    of lifesaving, 111–13
    shock and, 7–11
    see also ABCs
beaver fever, 143–47
bees, 123–24
Benadryl, 189
Bioclusive, 189
bites and stings, 115–35
    bee, 123–24
    blackfly, 123
    centipede, 125
    medicine kit for, 191
    millipede, 125
    mosquito, 122
    repellents and, 125–26
    reptile, 135
    scorpion, 120–21
    snake, 127–35
    spider, 115–19
blackflies, 123
black widow spiders, 116–17
blast effect, of lightning, 102, 104
bleeding:
    intracranial, 50–52
    see also blunt injuries; penetrating injuries; wounds
blindness, snow, 65–66
blisters, 176–77
blood clots, on brain, 50–52
blunt injuries:
    to abdomen, 61–62
    to chest, 56–59
    to eyes, 65
    see also soft-tissue injuries
body position sensors, seasickness and, 152
Borrelia burgdorferi, 163
brackish water, 111
breastbone, 57
breathing:
    in CPR, 15
    head and neck injuries and, 48
    lightning injury and, 105
    postimmersion syndrome and, 114
    in shock, 10
broken dentures, 175
brown spiders, 118–19
buboes, 161
buddy splints, 21, 39
burning/tanning characteristics, 88, 90
burns, 28–33
    feathering, 103
    severity of, 29–31
    types of, 32–33

Calamine, 190
calluses, 177
cancer, skin, 91
cardiac arrest, from lightning, 103
cardiopulmonary resuscitation, *see* CPR
cartilage, separated, 57
Cavit, 190
centipedes, 125
Centruroides exilicauda, 120–21
cerebral edema, high-altitude (HACE), 169
charcoal, granular activated, 148
chemical burns, 32
chest, 54–60
  flail, 57–58
  penetrating injuries to, 59–60
  sucking injuries to, 59–60
chilblains, 86
choking, 11–13, 69–70
circulation:
  in drowning, 114
  in fractures, 35
  head and neck injuries and, 48
  lightning injury and, 104, 105
  in shock, 10–11
citronella, 126
clothing:
  hypothermia prevented by, 75–76, 78–79
  solar injuries prevented by, 92
CMS (circulation, motor function, and sensation), 35, 37,
    41, 43
cock-up splint, 38
cold:
  injuries caused by, 86
  survival in, 179–82
  see also frostbite; hypothermia
collarbone fractures, 37
Colorado tick fever, 165
compression, in sprain treatment, 20
concussion, 50
conduction, heat loss and, 72
contact injury, from lightning, 102
contact lenses, 66–67
contusions, 21–22
convection, heat loss and, 72
copperhead snakes, 130
coral snakes, 128–29, 133
cornea:
  abrasions and foreign bodies in, 63–65
  frozen, 66
  sunburn of, 65–66
corns, 177
cottonmouth snakes, 130
CPR (cardiopulmonary resuscitation):
  ABCs in, 15–16
  for drowning, 114
  for hypothermia, 75, 80

CPR (cardiopulmonary resuscitation) *(cont.)*
   for lightning injury, 100, 105
   for shock, 10, 15–17
cramps, heat, 94–95
crepitus, 19, 35, 41
crowns, of teeth, 172, 175
Cyclizine, 154
cysts, 144
Decadron, 190
deep frostbite, 83–84
Deet, 125, 126
dental emergencies, 171–75
   infections in, 174–75
   toothaches in, 172–74
   trauma in, 175
dental infections, 174–75
   acute apical abscess, 174
   deep, 174–75
   pericoronitis, 174
   periodontal abscess, 174
dentin, 172
dentures, broken, 175
dermatitis, plant, 136–42
desert survival, 185–86
detached retina, 65
diamondback rattlesnakes, 128, 131
diarrhea, infectious, 143–47
Dimenhydrinate, 154
dimethylphthalate, 126
Diphenhydramine, 190
dislocation, 42–45
   of elbow, 44
   of finger, 45
   of hip, 45
   of kneecap, 45
   of retina, 65
   of shoulder, 43–44
dizziness, ear disorder and, 68
Domeboro tablets, 190
Donnagel, 187, 190
dramamine, 190
dressing pads, 188
drowning and near-drowning, 108–14
   lifesaving and treatment for, 111–14
   physiology of, 109–10
drugs:
   drowning caused by, 109
   hypothermia caused by, 74
dry drowning, 110
Eardrum, ruptured, 68–69
ears, 67–69
   dizziness and, 68
   lightning's effect on, 104
   swimmer's, 67–68
eastern diamondback rattlesnakes, 128, 131

edema:
  heat, 95
  high-altitude cerebral, 169
  high-altitude pulmonary, 169–70
elastic bandages, 191
elbows:
  dislocated, 44
  fractured, 38
electrical burns, 33
electromagnetic spectrum, 87–88
elevation, in sprain treatment, 20
enamel, 172
epidural hematoma, 50–52
eschar, 83
esophagus, 69–70
evacuation risks, in head injury, 52–53
evaporation, heat loss and, 72
exertional heat illnesses, 96–97
exhaustion, heat, 95–96
exposure to elements:
  hypothermia related to, 73
  solar injuries related to, 91
eye movements, in head and neck injuries, 48
eyes, 63–67
  blunt injuries to, 65
  contact lenses and, 66–67
  corneal foreign bodies and abrasions in, 63–65
  lighting's effect on, 104
  snow blindness, 65–66
  solar retinitis, 66
  sunglasses and, 67
Feathering burns, 103
fiberglass, as electrical insulator, 107
filters, for water, 148
finger, dislocated, 45
finger sweep, 13
fire, without matches, 182
first-aid kit, for wilderness, 192
fish hook removal, 25–26
flail chest, 57–58
flaps, skin, 23, 25
flashover effect, of lightning, 102–3
flatus expulsion, high-altitude (HAFE), 170
food, in wilderness survival, 182–83, 186
foot:
  athlete's, 178
  blisters on, 176–77
  calluses on, 177
  corns on, 177
  fractured, 42
  ingrown toenails on, 178
  trench, 86
forearm fractures, 38
foreign bodies, corneal, 63–65
foreign body granulomas, 137

fractures, 19, 34–42
  breastbone, 57
  evaluation of, 35–36
  pelvis, 40–41
  rib, 56–57
  spine and lower extremity, 39–42
  splints and slings for, 37, 38, 39, 40–42
  thighbone, 40–41
  tooth, 175
  upper arm, 38
  upper extremity, 37–39
Francisella tularensis, 161–62
fresh water aspiration, 110
friction burns, 33
frostbite, 81–86
  prevention of, 85–86
  treatment of, 84
  types of, 83–84
frostnip, 83
frozen cornea, 66
full-thickness avulsions, 24
full-thickness burns, 30
Giardia lamblia, 143–46, 148
Gila monsters, 135
granular activated charcoal, 148
granulomas, foreign body, 137
ground current, of lightning, 102
group therapy, for lightning injury, 105–6
HACE (high-altitude cerebral edema), 169
HAFE (high-altitude flatus expulsion), 170
halogens, 148
hand fractures, 39
HAPE (high-altitude pulmonary edema), 169–70
HDCV (human diploid cell vaccine), 159
head and neck injuries, 47–53
  ABCs of treatment of, 48–49
  drowning caused by, 109
  evacuation risks in, 52–53
  types of, 50–52
head-tilt technique, 15
heat cramps, 94–95
heat edema, 95
Heat Escape Lessening Posture (HELP), 79
heat exhaustion, 95–96
heat illness, 93–97
  cramps in, 94–95
  edema in, 95
  exertional, 96–97
  exhaustion in, 96
  prevention of, 98
  sunstroke in, 97
  syncope in, 95
  see also sun
heatstroke, 97
Heimlich maneuver, 12–14, 114
HELP (Heat Escape Lessening Posture), 79

hematomas:
    subdural, 50–51
    subungual, 22
hemothorax, 59
high-altitude illness, 166–70
    cerebral edema, 169
    flatus expulsion, 170
    mountain sickness, 167–69
    pulmonary edema, 169–70
hip:
    dislocated, 45
    fractured, 40–41
honeybees, 123, 124
hornets, 123
HRIG (human rabies immune globulin), 159
human diploid cell vaccine (HDCV), 159
"hydrophobia," in rabies, 158
hydrotherapy, 21
Hymenoptera, 123
hypertonicity, 110–11
hyperventilation, drowning caused by, 109
hyphema, 65
hypothermia, 71–80
    causes of, 71–74
    CPR and, 75, 78
    drowning and, 109
    immersion, 77–80
    types of, 74
hypotonicity, 110
Ice, in sprain treatment, 20
immersion, 108, 111
immersion foot, 86
immersion hypothermia, 77–80
immobility, hypothermia caused by, 73–74
infectious diarrhea, 143–47
ingrown toenails, 178
insect repellents, 125–26
insect sting kits, 191
intracranial bleeding, 50–52
Ixodes ticks, 163
"Jaw-thrust" technique, 10
Keratoses, solar, 91
Kerlix roll bandages, 188
Kling roll bandages, 188
kneecap:
    dislocated, 45
    fractured, 41
Labyrinthitis, 68
lacerations, 23–24
    see also specific body parts
Latrodectus mactans, 116–17
leader stroke, in lightning, 101
lenses:
    contact, 66–67
    for sunglasses, 67
Leptospira icterohaemorrhagiae, 162

leptospirosis, 162–63
lifesaving, basic, 111–13
ligaments, torn, 19
lightning, 99–107
    avoiding injuries from, 106–7
    forms of, 101
    injuries from, 102–4
    myths and superstitions about, 99–100
    treatment of injuries from, 104–5
lizards, 135
Lomotil, 190
loose teeth, 175
lower leg fractures, 41
Loxosceles spiders, 118–19
Lycosidae, 119
Lyme disease, 163–64
Major burns, 30–31
malignant melanoma, 91
Massasauga rattlesnakes, 131
Meclizine, 154, 189
medical kit, wilderness, 187–92
    first-aid materials for, 192
    miscellaneous materials for, 190–92
    wound care materials for, 188–89
melanin, 88
melanoma, malignant, 91
Miconazole cream, 190
mild hypothermia, 74–75
mild shock, 9
millipedes, 125
minor burns, 30
moderate shock, 9
mosquitoes, 122
motion sickness, 151–55
motor function:
    in fractures, 35
    head and neck injuries and, 48
mountain sickness:
    acute, 167–69
    mild, 167–68
MPD (myofascial pain-dysfunction) syndrome, 173–74
Near-drowning, *see* drowning and near-drowning
neck, *see* head and neck injuries
needlenose pliers, 191
nines, rule of, 30, 31
Northern Pacific rattlesnakes, 131
nosebleed, 69
Open wounds, 22–25
osteomyelitis, 35
Partial-thickness avulsions, 24
partial-thickness burns, 29–30
pearl lightning, 101
pelvis fractures, 40–41
penetrating injuries:
    in abdomen, 62
    in chest, 59–60

Pen VK, 190
periapical periodontitis, 173
pericoronitis, 174
periodontal abscess, 174
permethrin, 126
pernio, 86
phenergan, 190
pheromones, 123
photosensitivity, 90–91
physical fitness, hypothermia and, 78
phytophotodermatitis, 90
pilot stroke, in lightning, 101
pit vipers, 128–29
    see also snakes
plague, 160–61
plant dermatitis, 136–42
    allergic, 138–42
    primary irritant, 137–38
pneumothorax, 58
    tension, 55, 56, 58–59
poison ivy, 138–42
poison oak, 138, 139
poison sumac, 138, 139
postimmersion syndrome, 114
prairie rattlesnakes, 131
primary irritant dermatitis, 137–38
prodrome, in rabies, 158
Promenthazine, 154
pulled muscles, 21
pulmonary edema, high-altitude (HAPE), 169–70
pulp, dental, 172
pulpitis, 172
puncture wounds, 25–27
    fish hooks in, 25–26
    splinters in, 27
pygmy rattlesnakes, 128, 130–31
Rabies, 156–59
radiation, heat loss and, 72
rattlesnakes, 128, 130–31
reflectivity, 90
repellents, insect, 125–26
rest, in sprain treatment, 20
retina, 65
retinitis, solar, 66
ribbon lightning, 101
ribs, 56–57
RICE (rest, ice, compression and elevation), 20–21, 37, 42
Rocky Mountain Spotted Fever (RMSF), 164–65
rope burns, 33
rule of nines, 30, 31
ruptured eardrums, 68–69
Rutgers 612, 126
Safety pins, 191
St. Elmo's fire, 101, 106
Salmonella, 143, 146

Sawyer Extractor, for snakebite, 134, 191
Scopolamine, 154–55
scorpions, 120–21
seasickness, 151–55
seawater aspiration, 110–11
secondary drowning, 114
sedimentation, 147
seizures, drowning caused by, 109
separated cartilage, 57
separated shoulder, 44
severe hypothermia, 74–75
shallow-water blackout, 109
sheet lightning, 101
shelter:
   in cold weather, 180
   in desert, 185–86
Shigella, 143
shock, 7–11
shock position, 11
shoulder:
   dislocated, 43–44
   fractured, 37–38
   separated, 44
side flash, from lightning, 102
sidewinder snakes, 131
skin, 23, 24–25, 91, 188–89
   see also soft-tissue injuries
slings, 37
snakebite, 132–35
snakes, 127–35
snow blindness, 65–66
snow caves, 180
snow trenches, 180–81
SNS (sympathetic nervous system), 8
soap, 188
soft-tissue injuries, 18–27
   abrasions, 27
   contusions, 21–22
   open wounds, 22–25
   puncture wounds, 25–27
   sprains, 19–21
   strains, 21
   subungual hematomas, 22
   see also blunt injuries
solar injuries, *see* heat illness; sun
solar keratoses, 91
solar retinitis, 66
solar stills, 184
solar zenith angle, 89
Sonoran coral snake, 131
Southern Pacific rattlesnakes, 131
space heaters, burns from, 32
Spenco 2nd Skin, 189
SPF (sun protection factor), 92
spiders, 115–19
   black widow, 116–17

brown, 118–19
  tarantula, 119
  wolf, 119
spinal cord, 48–49
splash injury, from lightning, 102
splinter removal, 27
splints, 37
  buddy, 21, 39
  cock-up, 38
  for lower body fractures, 40–42
sprains, 19–21, 42
spray current, from lightning, 102
squamous cell carcinoma, 91
step voltage, of lightning, 102
sterile dressing pads, 189
stills:
  solar, 184
  vegetation, 184–85
stings, *see* bites and stings
strains, 21
streak lightning, 101
stride voltage, of lightning, 102
subdural hematoma, 50–52
submersion, 108
subungual hematomas, 22
sucking chest wounds, 59–60
sun, 87–93
  injuries caused by, 88–90, 91–92
  photosensitivity and, 90
  see also heat illness
sunburn, 93
sunglasses, 67
sun protection factor (SPF), 92
sunscreens, 92
sunstroke, 97
superficial frostbite, 83
superstitions, about lightning, 99–100
surfactant, 110, 111
Surgipads, 24, 188
survival, in wilderness, 179–86
  cold-weather, 179–82
  desert, 185–86
  food in, 182–83
  water in, 183–85
swimmer's ear, 67–68
sympathetic nervous system (SNS), 8
syncope, heat, 95
Tarantulas, 119
Tegaderm, 27, 189
tension pneumothorax, 55, 56, 58–59
Tetrahydrozoline, 190
throat, 69–70
thunder, 100–102
tick-related diseases, 163–65
timber rattlesnakes, 130
toenails, ingrown, 178

tongue blades, 191
tooth, fractured, 175
toothaches, 172–74
   MPD syndrome, 173–74
   periapical periodontitis, 173
   pulpitis, 172
torn ligaments, 19
tourniquets, 191
Transderm Scop, 154–55, 190
trauma:
   dental, 175
   see also shock
trench foot, 86
triangular bandages, 191
Trichophyton, 178
trophozoites, 144, 145
tularemia, 161–62
Tylenol No. 3, 190
Upper arm fractures, 38
urushiol, 140, 142
UVR (ultraviolet radiation), 65, 67, 87–91, 92
Vegetation stills, 184–85
venom, 132
verbal response, in head and neck injuries, 48
vestibular system, seasickness and, 152
vipers, 128–29
visual system, seasickness and, 152
Wasps, 123, 124
water, in wilderness survival, 183–185, 186
water disinfection, 147–50
water temperature, hypothermia and, 78
western coral snake, 131
western diamondback rattlesnakes, 131
wet drowning, 110
windburn, 90
wolf spiders, 119
wounds, 22–27
   materials for treatment of, 188–89
   open, 22–25
   puncture, 25–27
   sucking chest, 59–60
wrists, 20, 21, 38–39
Yellowjackets, 123, 124
Zinc oxide, 190